Allergic Contact Dermatitis

Editor

CHRISTEN M. MOWAD

DERMATOLOGIC CLINICS

www.derm.theclinics.com

Consulting Editor
BRUCE H. THIERS

July 2020 • Volume 38 • Number 3

ELSEVIER

1600 John F. Kennedy Boulevard • Suite 1800 • Philadelphia, Pennsylvania, 19103-2899

http://www.theclinics.com

DERMATOLOGIC CLINICS Volume 38, Number 3
July 2020 ISSN 0733-8635, ISBN-13: 978-0-323-71213-2

Editor: Lauren Boyle
Developmental Editor: Laura Kavanaugh

Dermatologic Clinics (ISSN 0733-8635) is published quarterly by Elsevier Inc., 360 Park Avenue South, New York, NY 10010-1710. Months of publication are January, April, July, and October. Business and editorial offices: 1600 John F. Kennedy Blvd., Suite 1800, Philadelphia, PA 19103-2899. Customer service office: 11830 Westline Drive, St. Louis, MO 63146. Periodicals postage paid at New York, NY, and additional mailing offices. Subscription prices are USD 408.00 per year for US individuals, USD 780.00 per year for US institutions, USD 456.00 per year for Canadian individuals, USD 952.00 per year for Canadian institutions, USD 510.00 per year for international individuals, USD 952.00 per year for international institutions, USD 100.00 per year for US students/residents, USD 100.00 per year for Canadian students/residents, and USD 240 per year for international students/residents. International air speed delivery is included in all *Clinics* subscription prices. All prices are subject to change without notice. **POSTMASTER:** Send address changes to *Dermatologic Clinics*, Elsevier Health Sciences Division, Subscription Customer Service, 3251 Riverport Lane, Maryland Heights, MO 63043. **Customer Service: 1-800-654-2452 (U.S. and Canada); 314-447-8871 (outside U.S. and Canada). Fax: 314-447-8029. E-mail: journalscustomerservice-usa@elsevier.com (for print support); journalsonlinesupport-usa@elsevier.com (for online support).**

Reprints. For copies of 100 or more, of articles in this publication, please contact the Commercial Reprints Department, Elsevier Inc., 360 Park Avenue South, New York, New York 10010-1710. Tel.: 212-633-3874; Fax: 212-633-3820; Email: reprints@elsevier.com.

The *Dermatologic Clinics* is covered in *MEDLINE/PubMed (Index Medicus)*, *Current Contents/Clinical Medicine, Excerpta Medica, Chemical Abstracts,* and *ISI/BIOMED.*

Contributors

CONSULTING EDITOR

BRUCE H. THIERS, MD
Professor and Chairman Emeritus, Department of Dermatology and Dermatologic Surgery, Medical University of South Carolina, Charleston, South Carolina

EDITOR

CHRISTEN M. MOWAD, MD
Professor and Director, Division of Dermatology, Geisinger Medical Center, Danville, Pennsylvania

AUTHORS

AMBER RECK ATWATER, MD
Associate Professor, Duke Dermatology, Durham, North Carolina

FRANCESCA Y BARUFFI, BS
MD Candidate, The George Washington School of Medicine and Health Sciences, Washington, DC

CHRISTOPHER CHU, MD
Dermatopathology Fellow, Department of Dermatology, Penn State Health, Milton S. Hershey Medical Center, Hershey, Pennsylvania

CORY A. DUNNICK, MD
Department of Dermatology, University of Colorado, Anschutz Medical Campus, Rocky Mountain Regional VA Medical Center, Aurora, Colorado

ALISON EHRLICH, MD, MHS
Dermatologist, Foxhall Dermatology, Washington, DC

ALEXANDRA FLAMM, MD
Assistant Professor, Department of Dermatology, Penn State Health, Milton S. Hershey Medical Center, Hershey, Pennsylvania

LAUREN CLAIRE HOLLINS, MD
Assistant Professor, Department of Dermatology, Penn State Health, Milton S. Hershey Medical Center, Hershey, Pennsylvania

SOPHIA HU, BA
University of Colorado School of Medicine, Aurora, Colorado

MATTHEW BARRETT INNES, MD
Tanner Clinic, Layton, Utah

SHARON E. JACOB, MD
Department of Medicine and Pediatrics, University of California, Riverside, Riverside, California; Department of Dermatology, Loma Linda University, VA Loma Linda, Loma Linda, California

MELISSA LAUGHTER, PhD
Rocky Vista University, College of Osteopathic Medicine, Parker, Colorado

JAMES G. MARKS Jr, MD
Professor, Department of Dermatology, Penn State Health, Milton S. Hershey Medical Center, Hershey, Pennsylvania

KARI MARTIN, MD
Department of Dermatology, University of
Missouri, Columbia, Missouri

MICHELLE MILITELLO, MS
Rocky Vista University, College of Osteopathic
Medicine, Parker, Colorado

SUSAN T. NEDOROST, MD
University Hospitals Cleveland Medical Center,
Professor of Dermatology, Case Western
Reserve University, Cleveland, Ohio

KAMARIA N. NELSON, MD, MHS
Research Fellow, Department of Dermatology,
The George Washington Medical Faculty
Associates, Washington, DC

SOLVEIG OPHAUG, MD
PGY-3 Resident Physician, Department of
Dermatology, Oregon Health & Science
University, Portland, Oregon

ALVA POWELL, BS
MD Candidate, The George Washington
School of Medicine and Health Sciences,
Washington, DC

MARGO J. REEDER, MD
Associate Professor, Department of
Dermatology, University of Wisconsin School
of Medicine and Public Health, Madison,
Wisconsin

DIANA M. SANTOS, BS
Medical Assistant, Department of
Dermatology, The George Washington
Medical Faculty Associates, Washington,
DC

KATHRYN SCHWARZENBERGER, MD
Professor, Department of Dermatology,
Oregon Health & Science University, Portland,
Oregon

MICHAEL P. SHEEHAN, MD, FAAD
Dermatology Physicians, Inc.,
Columbus, Indiana; Volunteer Faculty,
Department of Dermatology, Indiana
University School of Medicine, Indianapolis,
Indiana

ALLISON SINDLE, MD
Department of Dermatology, University of
Missouri, Columbia, Missouri

KAUSHIK P VENKATESH, BS
Graduate Clinical Research Student,
The George Washington School of
Medicine and Health Sciences, Washington,
DC

PEGGY A. WU, MD, MPH
Associate Professor, Department of
Dermatology, University of California, Davis,
Sacramento, California

Contents

Patch testing is the gold-standard diagnostic tool for the diagnosis of allergic contact dermatitis; unfortunately, it is a procedure with potential for errors, including false-negative reactions. Some of the factors responsible for this are likely unavoidable; however, others may potentially lie within the control of the user. Knowledge and management of these controllable factors may improve the outcome of patch testing and minimize the incidence of false-negative patch test results.

The duration of cutaneous inflammation preceding sensitization influences the resulting allergic response; the innate immune system instructs the adaptive immune response. Potent allergens that function as their own irritant cause classic T helper cell type 1 skewed dermatitis. Examples include poison ivy, epoxy resin, and methylchloroisothiazolinone. Less potent allergens, such as food proteins and propylene glycol, sensitize skin affected by chronic dermatitis resulting in a T helper cell type 2 skewed response, sometimes with associated systemic contact dermatitis. Systemic contact dermatitis should therefore be suspected in patients with positive patch tests to ingested allergens in the setting of chronic dermatitis.

Allergic contact dermatitis is a delayed type IV hypersensitivity skin reaction to external stimuli. Patterns of dermatitis depend on allergen exposure and patch testing is the gold standard to identify causal agents. The American Contact Dermatitis Society identifies an "Allergen of the Year" in order to highlight facts about particular allergens, which may range from showing increasing prevalence of disease, to documenting low levels of relevant allergic reactions. This article reviews the allergens of the year from 2000 to 2020 with an emphasis on clinical relevance. Categories of allergens include adhesives, dyes, medications, metals, preservatives, rubber accelerators, surfactants, and other skin care product ingredients.

Pediatric allergic contact dermatitis (Ped-ACD) is an increasingly recognized highly prevalent skin disease that has a significant impact on the quality of life of patients and their families. Accurate and appropriate patch testing is vital to diagnosing Ped-ACD. This requires knowledge of the most common allergens in the pediatric population, consideration of concurrent diseases that can complicate the clinical picture, and potential modification of techniques to lessen exposure to irritants and sensitizers while obtaining true positive results. This article reviews the most common pediatric allergens and discusses considerations when performing pediatric patch testing.

This article provides an overview of the evaluation and management of occupational contact dermatitis, including how to evaluate a patient with suspected occupational contact dermatitis. Patch testing, how to perform a site visit, and how to properly manage using preventative measures, prescribed therapies, and patient education are discussed.

The prevalence of occupational contact dermatitis is estimated to be between 6.7% and 10.6% and can lead to missed work and job loss. Although treatment may provide temporary relief, identifying the culprit allergen may help the clinician counsel on how to avoid or reduce exposure. Some of the most common high-risk occupations for allergic contact dermatitis include agricultural workers, construction workers, health care workers, hairdressers, mechanics, and machinists. In this article, we discuss the common occupational exposures of these high-risk professions, and summarize the common culprit allergens.

Education is the keystone of successful management of allergic contact dermatitis. This article outlines practical tips to manage patients' expectations of the patch test process and understand their results. The considerations are outlined in a stepwise fashion from before, during, and after patch testing. Resources for patient information are highlighted, and an update on provider education is also included.

Orthopedic implant hypersensitivity reactions (IHRs) are known to occur but are uncommon. Clinical presentations include local and generalized cutaneous reactions and noncutaneous complications. Pathogenesis traditionally was believed a type IV delayed hypersensitivity reaction, but there is evidence that innate immunity plays a role. Orthopedic implants are made predominantly of metals, and nonmetal components, such as bone cement, plastics, and ceramics, also may be utilized. Several diagnostic tests are available, and patch testing is considered the gold standard. Diagnostic criteria for IHRs have been developed and can help with determination as to whether orthopedic implant symptoms are due to IHRs.

Allergic contact dermatitis to fragrance is common. The prevalence of fragrance allergy in the general population is between 0.7% and 2.6%. In patch-test populations, the positive reaction rate to fragrances ranges from 5% to 11%. The most common fragrance screeners in most baseline series include fragrance mix 1, fragrance mix 2, and Balsam of Peru. The addition of hydroxyisohexyl 3-cyclohexene carboxaldehyde, hydroperoxides of limonene, and hydroperoxides of linalool to screening series can further aid in the diagnosis of fragrance allergy. In the proper clinical setting, supplemental patch testing with an additional fragrance or essential oil series should be considered.

DERMATOLOGIC CLINICS

SERIES OF RELATED INTEREST

Immunology and Allergy Clinics of North America
Available at: http://www.immunology.theclinics.com/

THE CLINICS ARE AVAILABLE ONLINE!
Access your subscription at:
www.theclinics.com

Preface
Contact Dermatitis Update

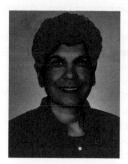

Christen M. Mowad, MD

Editor

Contact dermatitis is a stimulating field that impacts people of all races, genders, and ages. The study and diagnosis of allergic contact dermatitis (ACD) are filled with challenges that require knowledge, persistence, attention to detail, and curious inquiry. Each day we encounter hundreds of chemicals in the dozens of personal care products we contact. We are further exposed to numerous chemicals at work and in our avocations. Many of these chemicals have the potential to become allergens and cause chronic dermatitis. Considering the diagnosis of ACD is essential when evaluating patients with chronic dermatitis. Patch testing may be the step needed to identify the causative allergens, which may assist in resolution of the dermatitis.

One of the first patients I met in the patch-testing clinic was a plumber, who had suffered with hand dermatitis for nearly a decade. He had been treated with numerous topical and systemic medications without any relief. Patch testing resulted in 1 positive reaction to a chemical in the cleanser he used daily. Switching this simple cleanser resulted in complete resolution of his 10-year dermatitis. He was thrilled, and I was hooked.

Taking a detailed history of the presenting dermatitis, querying exposures the patient encounters at home and at work, allows the clinician to select the appropriate patient and allergens for patch testing, the criterion standard for diagnosing ACD. The goal of this testing process is to identify contact allergens that may contribute to, or exacerbate, dermatitis. Without considering ACD and choosing to patch test, the opportunity to identify a contact allergen may be missed. This may result in prolonged patient suffering, decreased quality of life, and unnecessary exposure to systemic immunosuppressive medications.

Contact allergy is a dynamic field. New allergens causing ACD are continually introduced into the marketplace, and many old allergens are repurposed. Being aware of new and repurposed allergens is critical to maintaining our ability to test with the most relevant allergens. Reviewing and adjusting screening series as new allergens are introduced into the marketplace is imperative in this process.

Once the diagnosis of ACD has been established and the causative allergens identified, education is paramount to the successful management of patient care. The multisyllabic words that identify these allergens can be challenging. Individuals diagnosed with ACD must be guided through the entire process from patch testing to allergen avoidance. Patients need to be educated on their allergies, including where they are found and how to avoid them. Databases can help patients identify products that are safe to use. Providers must engage patients with education and resources in order to ensure a successful patch-testing process, which requires a lifetime of allergen avoidance to maintain clearance.

Dermatol Clin 38 (2020) ix–x
https://doi.org/10.1016/j.det.2020.03.001

This issue of *Dermatologic Clinics* contains many topics central to ACD. I am hopeful that these articles will ignite a passion for contact dermatitis that those of us who have embraced patch testing as a subspecialty enjoy. The investigation, diligence, and patient education that are involved are extremely rewarding for both patient and provider. Identifying the causative allergen of a chronic dermatitis, engaging and helping the patient remove it from their environment, and watching chronic skin disease clear are satisfying for the clinician and life changing for the patient.

Christen M. Mowad, MD
Professor and Director, Division of Dermatology

Geisinger Medical Center, 16 Woodbine Lane
Danville, PA 17822, USA

E-mail address:
cmowad@geisinger.edu

Pitfalls in Patch Testing
Minimizing the Risk of Avoidable False-Negative Reactions

Solveig Ophaug, MD, Kathryn Schwarzenberger, MD*

KEYWORDS

- Patch testing • False-negative • Allergic contact dermatitis

KEY POINTS

- Patch testing for the diagnosis of allergic contact dermatitis can be complicated by both false-positive and false-negative results, some of which may be avoidable.
- Performing a delayed patch test reading is essential for valid results, and optimal results may be obtained by doing more than one delayed reading.
- Immunosuppressive therapies may suppress or diminish patch test responses.
- Newer immunomodulatory "biological" therapies have not yet been extensively studied but seem to potentially be safe for use during patch testing.
- Ultraviolet light in the area of patch testing before patch testing suppresses patch testing reactions.

INTRODUCTION

Patch testing is an imperfect science. Its successful use in the diagnosis of allergic contact dermatitis (ACD) is highly user dependent and involves many steps that can result in inconsistent or imperfect results. These begin with the choice of the patient being tested and includes the selection of test allergens, the concentration and vehicle of allergens used, the immune status of the patient, technical aspects of the procedure, interpretation and determination of the relevance of test results and, ultimately, patient education regarding these results. Both false-positive and false-negative results are possible outcomes, even in the hands of the most conscientious patch tester. False negatives in patch testing are by their nature difficult to identify and thus to quantify, so precise numbers as to their incidence are not readily available.

Colman is credited with having said that the greatest abuse of patch testing is not performing the test; however, arguably, obtaining a preventable false-negative result may be the second greatest sin.[1] Some of the factors known to be associated with false-negative results are technical and potentially beyond the immediate control of the patch tester, such as knowing (or having available) the optimal allergen concentration with which to test. Suboptimal handling of allergens may also result in a false-negative result; some allergens, including fragrances, acrylates, and other volatile substances, lose potency if loaded in the test chambers too far in advance of application.[2,3] Other factors, however, are more easily controlled by the patch tester, and some may have significant impact on the validity of the test results. One of the most important factors is ensuring that one or more delayed readings beyond the initial patch removal are performed. Another factor that can affect patch test results is the patient's immune status when testing. Patch testing assumes an intact immune system that can mount a delayed-type immune reaction in a patient previously

Neither Dr S. Ophaug or Dr K. Schwarzenberger report any relevant conflicts of interest.
Department of Dermatology, Oregon Health and Science University, 3303 SW Bond Avenue, CH16D, Portland, OR 97239, USA
* Corresponding author.
E-mail address: schwarka@ohsu.edu

Dermatol Clin 38 (2020) 293–300
https://doi.org/10.1016/j.det.2020.02.007
0733-8635/20/

sensitized to an allergen. Anything that affects the local or systemic immune system may compromise the ability to react to allergens during patch testing and potentially lead to false-negative results. These will be reviewed in detail here.

SUBOPTIMAL READING TIMES

Key points

- Single readings at the time of patch removal may result in both false-positive and false-negative reactions.
- Delayed readings are essential for detecting most of the positive reactions.
- Most true positive reactions will be evident by day 3 or 4.
- An additional day 7 reading may pick up additional significant reactions, particularly to metals, corticosteroids, and topical antibiotics.

The failure to perform a delayed reading is a well-appreciated and predictable cause of false-negative patch test reactions. Patch testing is designed to identify delayed-type hypersensitivity reactions, and, as such, involves a multiday testing procedure. Test allergens are applied on day 0, removed with a first reading after a defined period of time (a 2-day occlusion period is usually recommended),[4] and one or more delayed readings are performed a day or more later. Although some positive reactions may be evident at the time of patch removal on day 2, many do not fully develop until day 3 or later. Failure to perform readings beyond day 2 will miss these reactions. Rietschel and colleagues[5] noted that a single day 2 reading incurred an error rate as high as 56%, missing up to 34% of positive reactions that subsequently develop. They also showed that a significant number of apparent positive reactions at day 2, up to 22%, disappeared on subsequent reading and were likely irritant or false-positive reactions. Other studies confirmed that a single day 2 reading missed 20% to 40% of positive reactions.[6] A second reading between days 3 and 7 (72–168 hours) after initial patch application is thus essential to detect most of the allergic reactions. Most single delayed readings are performed on day 3 or 4 and, although different studies have favored 1 day over the other, neither has been shown to be clearly superior for detecting positive reactions.[7,8]

A second delayed reading (ie, third reading) beyond day 4 may increase the yield of positive reactions. Davis and colleagues[9] observed that delayed readings at day 5 detected most of the positive reactions, whereas readings at day 7 or later were useful in identifying reactions to metals and topical antibiotics. Of note, in their study, reactions to certain preservatives and fragrances dissipated after the day 5 reading and would have been missed with a single day 7 delayed reading. Similar studies have confirmed the value of performing a day 7 reading. Higgins and Collins identified new relevant day 7 positive reactions in 12.8% of their patients,[10] and more recently, in a large study involving more than 3000 patients, van Amerongen and colleagues found new positive reactions at day 7 in 13.6% of their patients.[11] Other studies have had similar outcomes.[12–14] The propensity to react late seems to be primarily a function of the allergen tested. Topical corticosteroids, metals, and neomycin frequently have late delayed reactions, as do some dyes (p-phenylenediamine and disperse dyes), acrylates, and some preservatives.[9,10,12–15] Patient characteristics have not been consistently found to affect patch test reactivity, although Torp Madsen and Andersen[14] did note more delayed reactions in women and patients older than 40 years. Similarly, the study by van Amerongen and colleagues[11] saw more late reactions in older individuals but noted that they could not completely rule out differences in sensitizing allergen exposure as a contributing factor. A prospective study in children with ACD found that 13% had new positive late delayed reactions at day 7 to 9.[16] No differences in delayed patch reactions have been noted between atopic and nonatopic dermatitis patients.[8,11] Further studies may be warranted to clarify if and to what extent age and other patient factors may affect the timing of patch test reactions.

The clinical scenario may help guide the choice to perform a second delayed reading. More allergies were detected in patients with oral lichenoid reactions when a day 7 reading was performed.[17] Given the propensity for metals to react late, day 7 readings are also appropriate when testing for implant-related allergies. Interpretation of positive reactions that develop beyond day 7 is tricky, as these may reflect newly acquired sensitization rather than a delayed reaction to an existing allergy.

The European Society of Contact Dermatitis guidelines for patch testing recommends 3 readings on day 2, day 3 or 4, and around day 7 as the optimal schedule.[4] Unfortunately, this schedule can be logistically challenging for both physicians and patients. They offer as an "acceptable" alternative schedule performing readings on day 2 and either day 3 or preferably day 4.[4] This schedule is used by many practitioners; however, the potential for missing a small percentage of late positive reactions should be acknowledged.

IMMUNOSUPPRESSION

The procedure of patch testing presumes a functional immune system with the ability to mount an allergic reaction to allergens to which the individual has been previously sensitized. ACD is a complex, incompletely understood process that has historically been thought to be driven primarily by a Th1-mediated immune response.[18] Th2, Th17, and Th22 immune responses are also involved, and recent work by Dhingra and colleagues[19] showed that different allergens might activate differential immune pathways. Their molecular profiling studies of ACD lesions found that nickel is a potent inducer of Th1 and innate immune responses but also activates Th17 and Th22 pathways, whereas fragrances and to a lesser extent, rubber, promotes primarily Th2 activity with some Th22 polarization, with much less Th1 and Th17 activity. Anything that might block these pathways or otherwise diminish cell-mediated immune responses could result in a false-negative reaction. The impact of systemic corticosteroids on patch testing has been relatively well studied; however, other immunosuppressant agents and newer immunomodulatory biologics have been less well investigated, with most information coming from case reports or small case series. In 2012, the North American Contact Dermatitis Group (NACDG) published recommendations on the use of immunosuppressive therapies during patch testing.[20] They acknowledged a paucity of experimental data about the impact of immunosuppressive therapies on patch testing and encouraged the performance of controlled, prospective studies. Unfortunately, 8 years hence, we have more drugs, but still relatively sparse data.

TOPICAL CORTICOSTEROIDS AND CALCINEURIN INHIBITORS

Key points

- Patch testing presumes an intact cell-mediated immune response.
- Both topical corticosteroids at the test site and oral corticosteroids have been shown to inhibit or diminish positive test results.
- The duration of inhibition by corticosteroids is not well defined.

Although there have been conflicting studies, recent or concurrent use of topical corticosteroids on the patch test site has been shown to diminish or impair allergic reactions in sensitized individuals and may result in false-negative results. In 1975, Smeenk demonstrated that application of topical triamcinolone 0.1% ointment for 24 hours before patch testing partially suppressed reactions in patient with nickel allergy.[21] The frequently cited study by Sukanto and colleagues[22] showed that topical application of corticosteroids for 24 hours before testing suppressed both the intensity and size of reactions to several contact allergens in sensitized individuals. Green similarly found that pretreatment with betamethasone dipropionate twice daily for 3 days suppressed or diminished both allergic and irritant reactions in most of the tested patients.[23] Conflicting reports included a study by Clark and Rietschel, in which they showed that triamcinolone 0.1% ointment applied 3 times daily for 1 week diminished patch test reactions in only a small minority of their patients.[24] Molander and colleagues[25] studied the question by injecting intralesional betamethasone into the patch test site for 3 days immediately before, during, and after patch testing; their protocol failed to suppress reactions to nickel.

Unfortunately, these studies are all relatively small and used different study protocols. It is perhaps notable in the study by Clark and Rietschel that the reactions that were diminished by corticosteroids were to formaldehyde or formaldehyde releasers (quaternium-15). It has not been clarified whether corticosteroids might have a differential impact on different allergens. The mechanisms by which corticosteroids exert their topical immunosuppressive effects are complex. Prens and colleagues[26] correlated diminished patch test response to topically applied corticosteroids in nickel-allergic patients with reductions in the number of Langerhans cells, activated inflammatory T cells, and mast cells. How long these effects persist in the skin has not been well studied. The NACDG consensus opinion was split with some experts recommending deferral of patch testing for 3 days and others 7 days after topical corticosteroid discontinuation.[20] Unfortunately, this can be difficult to accomplish in patients whose dermatitis involves their back.

Similar concerns have been raised about the potential for topical calcineurin inhibitors, tacrolimus, and pimecrolimus, to suppress patch test reactions; definitive studies are lacking to answer this question. One study in a small number of atopic dermatitis patients tested with the atopy patch test showed that pretreatment with pimecrolimus suppressed inflammatory reactions, whereas a similar study failed to show any suppressive effect from tacrolimus when compared with triamcinolone.[27,28] Additional studies are needed to clarify the impact these medications might have on patch testing; however, it seems prudent to consider the possibility that they might cause false-negative reactions.

SYSTEMIC CORTICOSTEROIDS

Early studies dating back to the 1950s confirmed that systemic corticosteroids might diminish or abrogate positive patch test reactions; Dr. Marion Sulzberger is credited with having been one of the earliest pioneers to report this potential impact.[29] Feuerman and Levy studied the effect of prednisone on the elicitation of positive patch tests to potassium dichromate and mercury. A daily 20 mg prednisone dose completely suppressed the reaction in only 6% of their patients, whereas higher doses decreased or completely inhibited reactions in significantly higher numbers.[30] O'Quinn in 1969 reported inhibition of positive patch test results in 6 of 20 patients treated with prednisone 40 mg daily.[31] In 1973, Condie and Adams demonstrated that daily administration of 40 mg/d for 7 days significantly diminished reactions to Rhus antigen.[32] Published recommendations in the early 2000s stated that patients on maintenance doses of systemic corticosteroids up to 20 mg daily could be patch tested without loss of significant reactions.[33] However, these findings were challenged in a more recent multicenter randomized, double-blind cross-over study by Anveden and colleagues,[34] which showed that prednisone 20 mg daily begun 48 hours before testing significantly decreased the total number of positive reactions to nickel sulfate; 25% of positive reactions were completely inhibited. Overall, the intensity of the positive reactions that did occur decreased, whereas prednisone had no impact on irritant reactions. They concluded that prednisone 20 mg/d does have a significant suppressive effect on allergic patch test reactions. Olupona and Scheinman subsequently published a case report of a patient who successfully reacted to multiple allergens when tested on prednisone 10 mg/d,[35] and Rosmarin and colleagues[36] similarly reported positive patch test results in several patients on lower dose prednisone (5–10 mg/d). Overall, these studies suggest that higher doses of systemic corticosteroids (>20 mg prednisone equivalent/day) may significantly interfere with successful patch testing, whereas positive results may still be elicited on lower doses (<20 mg/d prednisone equivalent). The NACDG consensus opinion states that although testing off corticosteroids is optimal, testing on 10 mg/d is acceptable.[20] Whether these lower doses potentially suppress weak results remains to be determined. The optimal duration off systemic corticosteroids

before testing remains uncertain and even among the NACDG experts, the recommended avoidance time ranged from 1 to 14 days.[20] Although most forms of oral corticosteroids are cleared from the blood fairly rapidly, their biological half-life, which is thought to correlate roughly with their antiinflammatory effect, is longer, and it is possible that antiinflammatory effect will persist longer than 7 days, particularly from the longer-acting corticosteroids, such as dexamethasone.[37] Thus we cannot reliably use drug half-life as a proxy for restoration of the immune system, as clearance of an immunosuppressive drug does not necessarily equal restoration of immune function.[38] The effects of intramuscular forms of triamcinolone last up to, or potentially even longer, than 4 weeks.

OTHER IMMUNOSUPPRESSIVE MEDICATIONS

Key points

- Systemic immunosuppressive medications may diminish or inhibit positive patch test responses and their use during patch testing is not recommended.
- Patch testing on methotrexate is thought to be acceptable, but confirmatory studies are small.
- Testing off all systemic therapies is optimal.

Systemic immunosuppressive therapies other than corticosteroids are thought to suppress patch test reactions, but relatively few studies have been done to determine the extent of problem. A study in the 1990s demonstrated that, in addition to controlling the underlying ACD, cyclosporine inhibited patch test reactions to different antigens.[39] Several studies since have shown that positive patch test reactions can be elicited in at least some patients on immunosuppressive medications. Wee and colleagues[40] prospectively patch tested 38 patients on chronic (≥1 month duration) therapy with immunosuppressive and/or immunomodulatory agents including azathioprine, cyclosporin, methotrexate, mycophenolatemofetil, adalimumab, infliximab, etanercept, and tacrolimus. At least one patient on each drug had a positive patch test reaction. Wentworth and Davis retrospectively evaluated 8 patients who underwent patch testing on immunosuppressive therapies (7 on methotrexate 7.5–30 mg/d, 1 on mycophenolatemofetil 1 gm daily). Four patients on methotrexate had one or more positive reactions. Most patients with positive reactions were on lower doses of methotrexate (<15 mg/wk).[41] The previously cited chart review by Rosmarin and colleagues[36] identified positive reactions in 11 patients on systemic immunosuppressants including prednisone, cyclosporine,

cyclosporine + prednisone, mycophenolatemofetil, and infliximab. All but one patient had reactions, 7 of which were strong or extreme reactions. One patient on mycophenolate reacted to cobalt, gold, and triethanolamine; when retested months later off mycophenolatemofetil, the patient reacted to multiple other allergens, including methylchloroisothiazolinone/methylisothiazolinone, diazolidinyl urea, DMDM hydantoin, and melamine formaldehyde. This suggests that mycophenolate did have a significant inhibitory effect on the patch testing. Several other case reports have reported positive patch test results in some of their patients taking immunosuppressants including methotrexate and azathioprine.[42–44]

In the absence of good studies to the contrary, these limited studies suggest that immunosuppressive drugs likely affect the ability to respond to patch tests. Methotrexate seems to have the least impact, leading the NACDG in their guidelines to suggest that it has "little to no effect", whereas others including azathioprine, cyclosporine and mycophenolatemofetil exert dose-dependent inhibition.[20] However, even when using methotrexate, the potential for a false-negative result cannot be ruled out. Whenever possible, testing should be postponed in patients who are on these medications and confirmatory testing off immunosuppressive therapy should be offered whenever possible.

TARGETED IMMUNOTHERAPIES

Key points

- Preliminary studies with dupilumab shows that although some reactions may be lost, positive reactions can be elicited.
- No inhibitory effect on patch testing has been demonstrated to date from immunotherapies targeting tumor necrosis factor alpha (TNF-α), interleukin (IL) 12/23, or IL-17.

Significant advances in the understanding of the pathogenesis of psoriasis and atopic dermatitis have been complemented by the development of targeted immunotherapies that block specific steps in the inflammatory processes. The potential impact of these immunomodulatory therapies on patch testing has been considered in recent studies.

DUPILUMAB

Although early studies suggested that dupilumab is likely safe to use during patch testing, its use remains somewhat controversial. Dupilumab is a monoclonal antibody that targets the IL-4 receptor α subunit, inhibiting signaling of IL-4 and IL-13. It is approved by the US Food and Drug Administration for treatment of moderate-to-severe atopic dermatitis and may benefit some patients when used off-label for the management of ACD.[45–54] This ability to suppress ACD led to concerns that dupilumab might also inhibit patch test responses. Several early case reports showed that patients on dupilumab could mount positive patch responses[55,56]; however, in subsequent reports, researchers found that although some positive reactions did occur on dupilumab, other responses were attenuated or lost.[57,58] Raffi and Botto proposed a possible allergen-specific response, which may correlate with different immune pathways preferentially activated by different allergens.[59] Stout and Silverberg patch tested 7 patients on dupilumab; although all had at least one positive result, one patient lost all previous positive reactions other than nickel.[52] Raffi and colleagues[57] recently did a large, retrospective analysis of patch test responses in 48 patients with atopic dermatitis treated with dupilumab. Twenty-three of these patients had patch testing done before initiation of dupilumab. When retested on dupilumab, 51.2% of positive responses were retained; however, 10.4% of responses were not reproduced or "lost" on dupilumab. The "lost" allergens included a wide range of allergens (fragrances, emulsifiers, sunscreens, nickel, and other preservatives). The investigators concluded that dupilumab does not uniformly diminish patch test results. Overall, these studies suggest that positive patch test results can be elicited in some patients on dupilumab. Although it is possible that underlying atopic dermatitis in many of these patients might confound the interpretation of patch test results and potentially lead to false-positive results, the finding that positive results may be attenuated or lost should be acknowledged when testing patients on dupilumab.

OTHER BIOLOGICS

TNF-α, IL-23, and IL-17 have been implicated in the pathogenesis of both ACD and psoriasis, and thus the potential for targeted therapies that block these molecules to inhibit sensitization and/or elicitation of ACD has been considered. Kim and colleagues[60] identified 15 psoriasis patients on biologics who underwent patch testing and compared them with a cohort of similar patients not on biological therapy. Drugs studied included the TNF-α antagonists infliximab, etanercept, and adalimumab, as well as the IL-12/23 blocker ustekinumab. They found no significant differences in the ability to react to patch tests among the co-horts, with reactions ranging from mild to robust over a relatively wide range of different allergens. However, the number of patients studied was small and, without confirmatory testing before or after use of the medication, it is not possible to state that all potential reactions were elicited on therapy. However, this study did demonstrate that positive patch reactions can occur while on targeted immunotherapies. Several case reports and small case series have similarly found positive patch results in patients on biologics including eta-nercept, adalimumab, infliximab, ustekinumab, and secukinumab.[36,40,41,60–62]

ULTRAVIOLET LIGHT

- Ultraviolet (UV) light on the skin exerts both local and systemic immunosuppressive effects.
- UV exposure to the area of patch testing before patch testing may inhibit patch test responses.
- There is no universally agreed on time for UV avoidance before patch testing.

The immunosuppressive effect of UV radiation on the skin is well established, and, although numerous studies have explored the mechanisms by which it is induced, only 2 studies have specif-ically examined the impact of UV light on patch test results in humans. Sjövall and Christensen performed patch testing on 9 patients with patch-test–positive nickel hypersensitivity before and after a course of UVB phototherapy given 4 times weekly for 3 weeks. Patch test reactions were significantly decreased in both frequency and intensity on both UV exposed and nonex-posed skin, suggesting that UV radiation has both local and generalized immunosuppressive ef-fects.[63] Notably, the investigators saw no signifi-cant difference in the frequency or intensity of allergic reactions when the protocol was repeated with exposure to UVA. In the other study, Daunton and Williams[64] retrospectively compared rates of positive patch test reactions between a small cohort of patients who had received phototherapy in the preceding 6 weeks and controls who had not. They found no significant difference between the 2 groups and concluded that cutaneous immu-nosuppression induced by UV exposure seems to fully resolve in less than 6 weeks.

Current North American and international guidelines recommend delaying patch testing af-ter exposure to natural or artificial UV light, as UV-induced cutaneous immunosuppression may result in false-negative reactions. Unfortunately,

these guidelines are primarily opinion based, and evidence regarding the amount of UV expo-sure and ideal time interval between exposure and patch testing is limited. The British Associa-tion of Dermatologists recommends deferring patch testing for at least 6 weeks after UV expo-sure, acknowledging that this timeframe is based on expert opinion.[65] The NACDG counsels avoid-ance of UV radiation for 1 week (range 0 days to 2 weeks) before patch testing.[20] The European Society of Contact Dermatitis guidelines suggest "postponing" patch testing but do not offer specific time recommendations.[4] These different recommendations highlight the need for further studies to better clarify the duration of immunosuppression in the skin by UV radiation. In the meantime, the likely impact of both tanning (indoor or artificial) and photother-apy must be considered when performing patch testing.

SUMMARY

False-negative patch test results are not completely avoidable, but those that can be, should be. Performance of delayed patch test readings is essential to detect positive reactions, and a second delayed reading at day 7 may opti-mize results. Failure to perform delayed readings will almost certainly produce false-negative re-sults. Anything that alters the patient's immune system and ability to mount a delayed-type hy-persensitivity reaction might affect their ability to react to patch tests. False-negative results may occur if patients tested have recently used topical or systemic corticosteroids, have had UV light exposure on their backs, or are on systemic immunosuppressive medications. Additional studies are warranted to clarify if and to what extent newer biological drugs may have on patch test reactions.

REFERENCES

1. Colman C. The use and abuse of patch testing. In: Maibach H, Gollin G, editors. Occupational and in-dustrial dermatology. Chicago: Mosby; 1982. p. 131–2.
2. Mowitz M, Svedman C, Zimerson E, et al. Fragrance patch tests prepared in advance may give false-negative reactions. Contact Dermatitis 2014;71(5): 289–94.
3. Gilpin SJ, Hui X, Maibach HI. Volatility of fragrance chemicals: patch testing implications. Dermatitis 2009;20(4):200–7.
4. Johansen JD, Aalto-Korte K, Agner T, et al. Euro-pean Society of Contact Dermatitis guideline for

diagnostic patch testing - recommendations on best practice. Contact Dermatitis 2015;73(4):195–221.

5. Rietschel RL, Adams RM, Maibach HI, et al. The case for patch test readings beyond day 2.Notes from the lost and found department. J Am AcadDermatol 1988;18(1 Pt 1):42–5.

6. Shehade SA, Beck MH, Hillier VF. Epidemiological survey of standard series patch test results and observations on day 2 and day 4 readings. Contact dermatitis 1991;24(2):119–22.

7. Todd DJ, Handley J, Metwali M, et al. Day 4 is better than day 3 for a single patch test reading. Contact Dermatitis 1996;34(6):402–4.

8. Geier J, Gefeller O, Wiechmann K, et al. Patch test reactions at D4, D5 and D6. Contact Dermatitis 1999;40(3):119–26.

9. Davis MDP, Bhate K, Rohlinger AL, et al. Delayed patch test reading after 5 days: The Mayo Clinic experience. J Am AcadDermatol 2008;59(2):225–33.

10. Higgins E, Collins P. The relevance of 7-day patch test reading. Dermatitis 2013;24(5):237–40.

11. van Amerongen CCA, Ofenloch R, Dittmar D, et al. New positive patch test reactions on day 7—The additional value of the day 7 patch test reading. Contact Dermatitis 2019;81(4):1–8.

12. Macfarlane AW, Curley RK, Graham RM, et al. Delayed patch test reactions at days 7 and 9. Contact dermatitis 1989;20(2):127–32.

13. Jonker MJ, Bruynzeel DP. The outcome of an additional patch-test reading on days 6 or 7. Contact Dermatitis 2000;42(6):330–5.

14. Torp Madsen J, Andersen KE. Outcome of a second patch test reading of TRUE Tests® on D6/7. Contact Dermatitis 2013;68(2):94–7.

15. Isaksson M. Corticosteroid contact allergy–the importance of late readings and testing with corticosteroids used by the patients. Contact dermatitis 2007;56(1):56–7.

16. Matiz C, Russell K, Jacob SE. The importance of checking for delayed reactions in pediatric patch testing. PediatrDermatol 2011;28(1):12–4.

17. Ahlgren C, Isaksson M, Möller H, et al. The necessity of a test reading after 1 week to detect late positive patch test reactions in patients with oral lichen lesions. Clin Oral Investig 2014;18(5):1525–31.

18. Gaspari AA, Katz SI, Martin SF. Contact hypersensitivity. CurrProtocImmunol 2016;113:4.2.1–4.2.7.

19. Dhingra N, Shemer A, Correa da Rosa J, et al. Molecular profiling of contact dermatitis skin identifies allergen-dependent differences in immune response. J Allergy ClinImmunol 2014;134(2):362–72.

20. Fowler JFJ, Maibach HI, Zirwas M, et al. Effects of immunomodulatory agents on patch testing: expert opinion 2012. Dermatitis 2012;23(6):301–3.

21. Smeenk G. Influence of local triamcinolone acetonide on patch test reactions to nickel sulfate. Dermatologica 1975;150(2):116–21.

22. Sukanto H, Nater JP, Bleumink E. Influence of topically applied corticosteroids on patch test reactions. Contact dermatitis 1981;7(4):180–5.

23. Green C. The effect of topically applied corticosteroid on irritant and allergic patch test reactions. Contact dermatitis 1996;35(6):331–3.

24. Clark RA, Rietschel RL. 0.1% triamcinolone acetonide ointment and patch test responses. Arch Dermatol 1982;118(3):163–5.

25. Molander G, Petman L, Kannas L, et al. Single doses of local betamethasone do not suppress allergic patch test reactions to nickel sulfate. Contact dermatitis 2004;50(4):218–21.

26. Prens EP, Benne K, Geursen-Reitsma AM, et al. Effects of topically applied glucocorticosteroids on patch test responses and recruitment of inflammatory cells in allergic contact dermatitis. Agents Actions 1989;26(1–2):125–7.

27. Weissenbacher S, Traidl-Hoffmann C, Eyerich K, et al. Modulation of atopy patch test and skin prick test by pretreatment with 1% pimecrolimus cream. Int Arch Allergy Immunol 2006;140(3):239–44.

28. Oldhoff JM, Knol EF, Laaper-Ertmann M, et al. Modulation of the atopy patch test: tacrolimus 0.1% compared with triamcinolone acetonide 0.1%. Allergy 2006;61(5):622–8.

29. Sulzberger MB, Witten VH, Zimmerman EH. The effects of oral cortisone acetate on patch test reactions to eczematogenous contact allergens. ActaDermVenereolSuppl (Stockh) 1952;32(29):343–52.

30. Feuerman E, Levy A. A study of the effect of prednisone and an antihistamine on patch test reactions. Br J Dermatol 1972;86(1):68–71.

31. O'Quinn SE, Isbell KH. Influence of oral prednisone on eczematous patch test reactions. Arch Dermatol 1969;99(4):380–9.

32. Condie MW, Adams RM. Influence of oral prednisone on patch-test reactions to Rhus antigen. Arch Dermatol 1973;107(4):540–3.

33. Rietschel RL, Fowler JFJ. Practical aspects of patch testing. In: Rietschel RL, Fowler JFJ, editors. Fisher's contact dermatitis. 5th edition. Philadelphia: Lippincott, Williams and Wilkins; 2001. p. 13.

34. Anveden I, Lindberg M, Andersen KE, et al. Oral prednisone suppresses allergic but not irritant patch test reactions in individuals hypersensitive to nickel. Contact dermatitis 2004;50(5):298–303.

35. Olupona T, Scheinman P. Successful patch testing despite concomitant low-dose prednisone use. Dermatitis 2008;19(2):117–8.

36. Rosmarin D, Gottlieb AB, Asarch A, et al. Patch-testing while on systemic immunosuppressants. Dermatitis 2009;20(5):265–70.

37. Becker DE. Basic and clinical pharmacology of Glu-cocorticosteroids. AnesthProg 2013;60(1):25–32.

38. Fauci AS, Dale DC, Balow JE. Glucocorticosteroid therapy: mechanisms of action and clinical consid-erations. Ann Intern Med 1976;84(3):304–15.

39. Higgins EM, McLelland J, Friedmann PS, et al. Oral cyclosporin inhibits the expression of contact hyper-sensitivity in man. J Dermatol Sci 1991;2(2):79–83.

40. Wee JS, White JML, McFadden JP, et al. Patch testing in patients treated with systemic immunosup-pression and cytokine inhibitors. Contact dermatitis 2010;62(3):165–9.

41. Wentworth AB, Davis MDP. Patch testing with the standard series when receiving immunosuppressive medications. Dermatitis 2014;25(4):195–200.

42. Verma KK, Bhari N, Sethuraman G. Azathioprine does not influence patch test reactivity in Parthenium dermatitis. Contact Dermatitis 2016;74(1):64–5.

43. Pigatto PD, Cesarani A, Barozzi S, et al. Positive response to nickel and azathioprine treatment. J EurAcadDermatolVenereol 2008;22(7):891.

44. Yfanti I, Nosbaum A, Berard F, et al. Methotrexate does not impede the development of contact allergy. Contact Dermatitis 2018;78(3):223–4.

45. Jacob SE, Sung CT, Machler BC. Dupilumab for sys-temic allergy syndrome with dermatitis. Dermatitis 2019;30(2):164–7.

46. Sung CT, McGowan MA, Machler BC, et al. Systemic treatments for allergic contact dermatitis. Dermatitis 2019;30(1):46–53.

47. Machler BC, Sung CT, Darwin E, et al. Dupilumab use in allergic contact dermatitis. J Am AcadDerma-tol 2019;80(1):280–1.e1.

48. Joshi SR, Khan DA. Effective use of dupilumab in managing systemic allergic contact dermatitis. Dermatitis 2018;29(5):282–4.

49. Chipalkatti N, Lee N, Zancanaro P, et al. A retrospective review of dupilumab for atopic dermatitis patients with allergic contact dermatitis. J Am AcadDermatol 2019;80(4):1166–7.

50. Chipalkatti N, Lee N, Zancanaro P, et al. Dupilumab as a treatment for allergic contact dermatitis. Dermatitis 2018;29(6):347–8.

51. Yang EJ, Murase JE. Recalcitrant anal and genital pruritus treated with dupilumab. Int J WomensDer-matol 2018;4(4):223–6.

52. Stout M, Silverberg JI. Variable impact of dupilumab on patch testing results and allergic contact dermatitis in adults with atopic dermatitis. J Am AcadDermatol 2019;81(1):157–62.

53. van der Schaft J, Thijs JL, de Bruin-Weller MS, et al. Dupilumab after the 2017 approval for the treatment of atopic dermatitis: what's new and what's next? CurrOpin Allergy ClinImmunol 2019;19(4):341–9.

54. Goldminz AM, Scheinman PL. A case series of dupilumab-treated allergic contact dermatitis pa-tients. DermatolTher 2018;31(6):e12701.

55. Hoot JW, Douglas JD, Falo LDJ. Patch testing in a patient on dupilumab. Dermatitis 2018;29(3):164.

56. Puza CJ, Atwater AR. Positive patch test reaction in a patient taking dupilumab. Dermatitis 2018;29(2):89.

57. Raffi J, Suresh R, Botto N, et al. The impact of dupi-lumab on patch testing and the prevalence of co-morbid ACD in recalcitrant atopic dermatitis: a retrospective chart review. J Am AcadDermatol 2020;82(1):132–8.

58. Zhu GA, Chen JK, Chiou A, et al. Repeat patch testing in a patient with allergic contact dermatitis improved on dupilumab. JAADCase Rep 2019; 5(4):336–8.

59. Raffi J, Botto N. Patch testing and allergen-specific inhibition in a patient taking Dupilumab. JAMADer-matol 2019;155(1):120–1.

60. Kim N, Notik S, Gottlieb AB, et al. Patch test results in psoriasis patients on biologics. Dermatitis 2014; 25(4):182–90.

61. Nosbaum A, Rozieres A, Balme B, et al. Blocking T helper 1/T helper 17 pathways has no effect on patch testing. Contact Dermatitis 2013;68(1):58–9.

62. Hamann D, Zirwas M. Successful patch testing of a patient receiving anti-interleukin-17 therapy with se-cukinumab: a case report. Contact Dermatitis 2017; 76(6):378–9.

63. Sjovall P, Christensen OB. Local and systemic effect of ultraviolet irradiation (UVB and UVA) on human allergic contact dermatitis. ActaDermVenereol 1986;66(4):290–4.

64. Daunton A, Williams J. The impact of ultraviolet expo-sure on patch testing in clinical practice: a case–control study. ClinExpDermatol 2019;45(1):25–9.

65. Johnston GA, Exton LS, MohdMustapa MF, et al. British Association of Dermatologists' guidelines for the management of contact dermatitis 2017. Br J Dermatol 2017;176(2):317–29.

Allergic Contact Sensitization in Healthy Skin Differs from Sensitization in Chronic Dermatitis
Atopic, Occupational Wet Work, and Stasis Dermatitis

Susan T. Nedorost, MD

KEYWORDS

- Allergic contact dermatitis • Atopic dermatitis • Systemic contact dermatitis • Food allergy
- Protein contact dermatitis • Occupational hand dermatitis • Stasis dermatitis
- Cutaneous microbiome

KEY POINTS

- In a patient with previously healthy skin, ask about exposure to potent allergens, or acute exposures causing irritation leading to sensitization (eg, spilling biocide on the skin at high concentration).
- In a patient with chronic dermatitis such as hand dermatitis owing to wet work or atopic dermatitis, consider testing for low potency allergens such as foods, tocopherol acetate, lanolin, and propylene glycol.
- In a patient with chronic dermatitis and failure to clear after contact avoidance of identified contact allergens, consider systemic contact dermatitis.
- In a patient with chronic dermatitis, consider sensitization to commensal organisms, which may occur in biofilms in patients with atopic and stasis dermatitis.

INTRODUCTION

Dermatitis, also known as eczema, refers to a disrupted epidermis associated with an itchy inflammatory response. Allergic sensitization contributes to several phenotypes of dermatitis that are distinguished in part by variation in immunologic conditions at the time of sensitization (**Table 1**). There are several other factors that influence sensitization including traits of the allergen, such as molecular size and affinity for binding protein, concentration of the allergen per surface area of the exposed skin, and site of the epidermal surface first exposed. Environmental influences, such as the presence of UVB light at the time of initial exposure, and psychological stress can also influence sensitization.[1] This discussion will focus on the influence of the inflammatory status of the skin before sensitization and the resultant phenotype of dermatitis.

In healthy skin, allergic contact dermatitis occurs when a potent allergen (eg, poison ivy) contacts the skin. A single exposure results in an acute, delayed type hypersensitivity response producing allergic contact dermatitis with blisters that resolve over several weeks after a single exposure. Repeated intermittent exposures result in chronic allergic contact dermatitis with thickening and fissuring of the skin. The immune response in these cases is T helper cell type 1 (Th1) and is usually durable.[2]

University Hospitals Cleveland Medical Center, Case Western Reserve University, 11100 Euclid Avenue, Lakeside Suite 6223, Cleveland, OH 44106, USA
E-mail address: stn@case.edu

Dermatol Clin 38 (2020) 301–308
https://doi.org/10.1016/j.det.2020.02.006
0733-8635/20/

Table 1
Overview of the effect of cutaneous inflammation on allergic contact sensitization

	Allergic Contact Dermatitis in Healthy Patients	Allergic Contact Dermatitis in Patients with Chronically Inflamed Skin	Systemic Contact Dermatitis
Examples		Atopic dermatitis Occupational hand dermatitis in wet workers Stasis dermatitis	Delayed-type food allergy triggering atopic dermatitis
Potency of allergen in the local lymph node assay	Strong or extreme	Nonsensitizer or weak or moderate	Nonsensitizer or weak or moderate
T-cell profile	Th1	Th2	Th2
Duration of positive patch test status	Usually long (y)	Sometimes short (mo)	Unknown
Associated immediate type hypersensitivity	No	Sometimes	Often
Example allergens	Poison ivy; methylchlorois-othiazolinone; epoxy resin	Propylene glycol; tocopherol acetate	Balsam of Peru; foods; propolis; nickel
Effect of Th2 blockade, for example, dupilumab	Worsens	Improves	Improves

Abbreviations: Th1, T helper cell type 1; Th2, T helper cell type 2.

Sensitization in the setting of the chronic dermatitis of atopic dermatitis results in a Th1 response of shorter duration, with a more durable T helper cell type 2 (Th2) response.[2] Chronic inflammation also provides sufficient immune signal to allow less potent allergens, as defined by the local lymph node assay,[3] to sensitize.[4] Examples of these less potent allergens include propylene glycol, lanolin, parabens, foods, and commensal organisms. Chronic conditions predisposing to this type of sensitization with less potent allergens include atopic dermatitis owing to mutations in genes of the epidermal differentiation complex, occupational hand dermatitis in wet workers, and stasis dermatitis. Biofilms in the setting of chronic stasis dermatitis and atopic dermatitis may promote sensitization to commensal organisms.[5]

Chronic allergic contact dermatitis with Th2 skewing may be triggered by ingested or inhaled allergen exposure with homing of T cells to previous sites of allergic contact dermatitis. This condition is known as systemic contact dermatitis. Delayed type food allergy can be viewed as a form of systemic contact dermatitis.

THE EDUCATION OF T CELLS INFLUENCES THE PHENOTYPE OF DERMATITIS
Innate Immunity

Inborn immunity is not adapted to the environment, but rather is the result of evolutionary ability to recognize patterns of threat. Pattern recognition receptors (PRRs) may be secreted in response to a microbe or an injury and lead to recruitment of dendritic cells and T cells to begin an adaptive immune response. Defensins are examples of secreted PRRs.

Transmembrane PRRs are expressed on antigen–presenting cells. The Toll-like receptors are a group of transmembrane PRRs that, like the innate cytokine IL-1, lead to nuclear factor-κβ activation and link to the adaptive immune response.[6] Nuclear factor-κβ activation is necessary for skin dendritic cells to migrate to the regional lymph node and present antigen[7]

Immature dendritic cells capture antigens that pass through epithelial tight junctions. In childhood onset reactions (atopic dermatitis), there is decreased barrier efficacy of the stratum corneum and tight junction in the stratum granulosum, such that dendritic cells can access antigens in the epidermis.[8] These dendritic cells migrate to the regional lymph node where they mature and express antigens in cell surface major histocompatibility complexes. They go on to educate T cells in a manner that depends on several factors, including the initial innate response.

Influences on Adaptive Immunity

Education of T cells depends on the microenvironment and the timing of antigen exposure.[9] Healthy skin with normal lipids and keratinocytes and diverse commensal organisms maintaining the skin barrier, like the healthy gastrointestinal tract, is tolerogenic. A population of skin antigen presenting cells similar to intestinal antigen-presenting cells produces IL-10 and induces regulatory T cells.[10]

Early exposure to peanut is associated with tolerance,[11] suggesting that we should aim to establish tolerance early and before any chapping of skin that may increase the likelihood of initial immune exposure in the context of innate immune signals. The lower rate of peanut allergy in countries where initial exposure is with early consumption of peanut bambas,[12] as opposed to the United States, where exposure to peanut is often by self-feeding of peanut butter, suggests that food contact with perioral inflamed skin owing to drooling may play a role in peanut allergy.

T-cell response to a protein alone is short lived, but is enhanced by endotoxin as an adjuvant[13] that can induce IL-12 part 70, which amplifies a Th1 response. Presence of IL-4, IL-33, and thymic stromal lymphopoietin amplify the Th2 response[14] Recently, skin group 2 innate lymphoid cells, like Langerhans cells, have been shown to present antigen to T cells and to sense the presence of Staphylococcus aureus. Increased numbers of skin group 2 innate lymphoid cells are present in the skin of atopic dermatitis patients, where inflammation correlates with abundance of S

aureus.[15] Like other dendritic cells, Langerhans cell function varies with the microenvironment, and can either induce tolerance or allergy, depending on conditions at the time of sensitization.[16]

Micro-organisms as well as chemicals on the surface of the skin, and even skin components themselves such as lipid breakdown products of filaggrin[16] can influence innate immune response, which in turn influences the type of T cell that will be amplified by the adaptive immune response, for example, Th1, Th2, Th17, or T regulatory. Genetic predisposition to atopic dermatitis has been linked to filaggrin mutation in some cohorts.[17] This demonstrates the interplay of genetic influences on skin barrier, innate immune response, and T-cell response that determines the phenotype of allergic dermatitis. Epigenetic modifications add further complexity and are not yet fully understood.[18]

Chronic barrier inflammation may explain the changes that lead to Th2 skewed sensitization, including food allergy.[19]

The Atopic March: T Helper Cell Type 2 Cytokines Lead to Antigen-Specific IgE

IL-4 causes antigen presenting cells to create Th2 cells. T follicular helper cells in the lymph node produce IL-4 and help B cells to produce antigen-specific IgE.[20] This mechanism may explain the progression from atopic dermatitis to allergic rhinitis and asthma.[21]

Application of emollients to neonates at risk for atopic dermatitis beginning at birth and applied at least daily head-to-toe on all skin decrease the incidence of atopic dermatitis in infancy.[22] Those who do develop dermatitis have been shown to go on to develop food allergy such as to egg.[23]

The Microbiome in Dermatitis

Th2 cytokines decrease human beta-defensins, an innate antimicrobial peptide that also induces tight junction proteins. Reduced beta-defensins in atopic dermatitis decrease efficacy of the skin barrier and allow overgrowth of organisms like S aureus.[24]

Bacterial diversity is decreased in atopic dermatitis, with increased abundance of S aureus.[25] S aureus and Alternaria may form a biofilm,[26] increasing the concentration of Alternaria on inflamed skin. We speculate this may lead to Alternaria-triggered asthma in some patients. We have also found that Halomonas, a salt-loving bacteria that may also form biofilms in nature, may occur on human skin.[27]

Table 2
Potent allergens function as their own irritants and sensitize healthy skin

Source of Irritation	Example Allergen
Allergen functions as its own irritants	Poison ivy
Acute exposure to high concentration of allergen induces irritation	Spill of undiluted biocide containing methylchlorois-othiazolinine increases concentration in contact with the skin compared with that in coolant at usage concentration

PHENOTYPE 1: ALLERGIC CONTACT DERMATITIS IN PATIENTS WITH PREVIOUSLY HEALTHY SKIN

Innate signal is from the allergen itself with very potent allergens[3] (**Table 2**). Poison ivy, for example, is an allergen affecting a large percentage of the US population and is known to be both a strong irritant and allergen.[28] The irritant potential of a potent allergen is further increased in the context of a spill, where concentration of the allergen per area of skin is quite high. For example, a worker who spilled epoxy hardener into his shoe developed a contact allergy.[29]

When the allergen is of moderate potency, the patient will usually report some preexisting inflammation preceding the sensitization. This is the context in which secondary sensitizations develop (**Table 3**). When taking a history for allergic contact dermatitis in patients with previously healthy skin, inquire about irritant exposures that may predispose to sensitization.

Most standard patch test series consist of moderate to potent allergens, because they are composed based on the likelihood of sensitizing the general healthy population. The immune response to these allergens that occur in the context of strong, fairly acute irritation is usually Th1 skewed and lasts indefinitely. Patients should expect to require complete avoidance of these allergens for life.

There is rarely associated systemic contact dermatitis. Treatment with dupilumab will not decrease and will likely increase patch test reactivity to Th1 (potent) allergens such as methylisothiazolinone.[30] This author has seen a patient referred owing to worsening adult-onset dermatitis after treatment with dupilumab, who subsequently had positive patch tests to methylisothiazolinone and formaldehyde releasing preservatives and who cleared completely with allergen avoidance.

PHENOTYPE 2: ALLERGIC CONTACT DERMATITIS IN PATIENTS WITH CHRONICALLY INFLAMED SKIN

In these patients, the innate signal is owing to chronic cutaneous inflammation. This predisposes to Th2 skewing. Even potent allergens like dinitrochlorobenzene can cause Th2 skewing in patients with atopic dermatitis.[2] However, the sensitizer is more often only weakly potent or even a nonsensitizer in the local lymph node assay, as the chronic inflammation provides ample innate signal that is, prerequisite for sensitization. Isocyanate allergens have been shown to produce more Th2 cytokines on skin that has been irritated with tape stripping before sensitization[31] (**Table 4**).

When obtaining an exposure history in these patients, it is important to consider less common allergens that are often not part of the standard series. Topical medicaments applied to chronically inflammatory skin diseases are often sources of sensitization to components that are weak sensitizers. Propylene glycol and vitamin E are examples that are more prevalent in patients with atopic dermatitis than in the population without atopic dermatitis undergoing patch testing for dermatitis.[32] The weakly potent sensitizers parabens and lanolin are well-known examples in

Table 3
Moderately potent allergens sensitize in conditions of acute or subacute irritant dermatitis

Source of Irritation	Example Allergen
Skinned knee	Neomycin
Chapped skin in winter	Quaternium-15 as preservative in emollients

Table 4
Weakly potent allergens sensitize in the context of chronic inflammation, with Th2 skewing

Source of Irritation	Example Allergen
Atopic dermatitis	Propylene glycol
Hand dermatitis in wet workers	Food proteins
Stasis dermatitis	Lanolin, parabens

patients with stasis dermatitis.[33] Contact allergy to foods is reported exclusively in patients with atopic dermatitis and food handlers (occupational dermatitis in wet work).[34]

In some cases, patch testing near the site of dermatitis is needed to elicit a diagnostic patch test response.[35] This is true in stasis dermatitis, for example, where paraben patch tests may be positive only near the dermatitis on the leg, but not on the noninflamed skin of the back. Allergy to proteins such as tomatoes may manifest with both dermatitis and urticarial and systemic contact dermatitis.[36] Protein contact dermatitis is identified by atopy patch testing and may induce contact urticaria within 30 minutes and papular dermatitis 48 hours later. These tests may be more sensitive when performed near the presenting site of dermatitis, where patch tests may elicit vesicles.[37]

As noted elsewhere in this article, the microbiome is altered in chronic dermatitis. Allergic sensitization to commensal organisms can occur (**Table 5**). *Malaseezia*,[38] *Staphylococcus*, and *Candida*[39] are all recognized as cutaneous antigens.

The duration of the Th1 response is shortened in about two-thirds of patients with atopic dermatitis.[2] We do not know how to predict the duration or how often patch testing should be performed. The duration of Th2 response is much more durable in atopic dermatitis, and patients who develop immediate type allergy symptoms owing to downstream B cell production of antigen specific IgE may expect these symptoms to be long lasting.

Dupilumab is helpful in controlling dermatitis in these patients with Th2 skewed positive patch tests. Nickel has been shown to be capable of causing a Th2 skewed contact allergy response[40] as well as Th1 responses, the latter in a group of patients with allergic contact dermatitis not specified as having previously inflamed skin or atopic dermatitis.[41] A case series of patients with positive patch tests to nickel, fragrance, and the secondary surfactant cocoamidopropyl betaine reports improvement with dupilumab treatment.[42]

PHENOTYPE 3: SYSTEMIC CONTACT DERMATITIS—A SEQUELAE OF PHENOTYPE 2

In patients with sensitization to less potent allergens in the context of chronic dermatitis, exposure to the allergen triggers a Th2 response that can lead to both a T-cell–mediated response (including recall inflammation of an allergy patch test site) and an antigen specific urticarial response. When triggered by ingestion or inhalation, this mixed urticarial and eczematous response is called systemic contact dermatitis.

Systemic contact dermatitis often flares at the site of previous cutaneous elicitation, including the patch test site. Other areas of predilection are flexural and periorifical sites such as the eyelid and the anogenital region, as well as the lower back (**Fig. 1** shows a patient with involvement of the lower back owing to systemic contact dermatitis from propolis.)

Dyshidrotic hand eczema is sometimes a manifestation of systemic contact dermatitis. We have demonstrated intercellular deposits of IgG subtypes IgG1, IgG2, and IgG4 but not IgG3 on direct immunofluorescence of the skin from a patient with acute palmar and plantar blisters associated with tinea pedis (unpublished data David Soler PhD and the author, 2014). This finding is intriguing given multiple reports linking intravenous immunoglobulin therapy to onset of dyshidrotic eczema,[43]

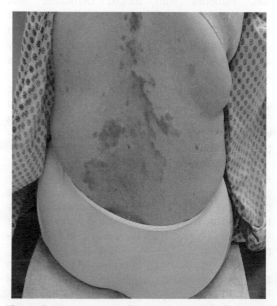

Fig. 1. Systemic contact dermatitis to propolis on the lower back.

Table 5	
Commensal organisms are weakly potent protein allergens that sensitize chronically inflamed skin	
Source of Irritation	**Example Antigen**
Atopic dermatitis with onset after puberty when sebum production allows growth	*Malaseezia sympodialis,* requiring oil for substrate
Atopic dermatitis in skin folds	*Staphylococcus* and *Candida*

and the possible implication of the IgG_1^+ memory B cells in perpetuating food allergy.[44]

Systemic contact dermatitis to methylparaben, confirmed by rechallenge, was described in a man with dermatitis of the interdigital webspaces of the hands, eyelids, buttocks, and thighs.[45]

A physician with eyelid dermatitis had a positive patch test to cinnamic alcohol and did not clear after avoidance of eye cosmetics, but cleared after avoiding cinnamon in foods and flared with rechallenge.[46] Several cases of systemic contact dermatitis to carmine have been described.[47] Systemic contact dermatitis to foods in the Liliaceae family including onion and garlic have been reported to cause both perioral, flexural, and lower back dermatitis[48] and dyshidrotic hand eczema.[49] Asparagus is also in this family[50]; the author recently had a patient with severe hand dermatitis and a positive patch test to diallyl disulfide, the allergen in onion and garlic, who flared after ingestion of asparagus.

The risk factors for systemic contact dermatitis are not well understood. Atopic dermatitis and wet work, in other words chronic cutaneous inflammation that often Th2 skews, seem to be risk factors for sensitization to allergens reported to cause systemic contact dermatitis. Examination of the author's own patch test database of more than 2000 patients, showed that children and adolescents with atopic dermatitis and respiratory atopy were more likely than age-matched patients with atopic dermatitis without respiratory atopy to have positive patch tests to 23 allergens previously reported to cause systemic contact dermatitis. Patients with atopic dermatitis with respiratory atopy and engaging in wet work, but not dry work, occupations were more likely than patients with atopic dermatitis without respiratory atopy to have positive patch tests to allergens known to cause systemic contact dermatitis.[51]

Not all sensitized patients develop systemic contact dermatitis. There is likely a requirement for homing of T cells to the cutaneous surface as well as Th2 skewing in dyshidrotic systemic contact dermatitis[52]

Systemic contact dermatitis should be considered in any patient who fails to clear completely after avoidance of an allergen identified by a positive patch test (**Table 6**). Systemic contact dermatitis to sorbic acid in foods has been reported after cutaneous sensitization to sorbic acid[53] and propylene glycol.[54]

Dupilumab has been of benefit to patients with systemic contact dermatitis owing to Balsam of Peru and nickel.[55] When atopic and allergic contact dermatitis are considered as separate disease states, the response to dupilumab is less clear.[56]

Table 6
In patients sensitized in the context of chronic cutaneous inflammation (atopic dermatitis or wet work), systemic avoidance of allergens is more likely to be necessary

Source of Sensitization	Example of Source of Systemic Contact Dermatitis
Contact allergy to sorbic acid in wipes in a young child	Foods containing sorbic acid
Medicament containing propylene glycol used on abrasions in a patient with a history of atopic dermatitis	Foods containing propylene glycol

Chronic irritant dermatitis owing to genetic barrier deficiency or wet work predisposes to Th2 skewing and systemic contact dermatitis. We are learning more about the less potent allergens that can sensitize patients, including commensal micro-organisms.

SUMMARY

Evaluation of dermatitis should include a detailed history to elicit whether worsening suggestive of allergic contact dermatitis occurred when skin was chronically inflamed or previously healthy. A broader group of less common (ie, less potent) allergens including protein allergens must be considered in patients sensitized in the context of chronically inflamed skin. This framework may improve value of care by identifying curative environmental modifications in some patients, and predicting response to expensive biologic drugs like dupilumab in others.

DISCLOSURE

The author has no commercial conflicts of interest; there was no funding source for this work.

REFERENCES

1. Rietschel R, editor. Fisher's contact dermatitis. 6th edition. Hamilton (Canada): BC Decker; 2008.
2. Newell L, Polak ME, Perera J, et al. Sensitization via healthy skin programs Th2 responses in individuals with atopic dermatitis. J Invest Dermatol 2013; 133(10):2372–80.

3. Gerberick GF, Ryan CA, Kern PS, et al. Compilation of historical local lymph node data for evaluation of skin sensitization alternative methods. Dermatitis 2005;16(4):157–202.

4. Kohli N, Nedorost S. Inflamed skin predisposes to sensitization to less potent allergens. J Am Acad Dermatol 2016;75(2):312–7.

5. Gonzalez T, Biagini Myers JM, Herr AB, et al. Staphylococcal biofilms in atopic dermatitis. Curr Allergy Asthma Rep 2017;17(12):81.

6. Flanklin Adkinson N, editor. Middleton's allergy: principles and practice. 8th edition. Philadelphia: Elsevier/Saunders; 2014. p. p2–19.

7. Baratin M, Foray C, Demaria O, et al. Homeostatic NF-κB signaling in steady-state migratory dendritic cells regulates immune homeostasis and tolerance. Immunity 2015;42:627–39.

8. Brandner JM, Zorn-Kruppa M, Yoshida T, et al. Epidermal tight junctions in health and disease. Tissue Barriers 2015;3(1–2):e974451.

9. Novak N, Koch S, Allam JP, et al. Dendritic cells: bridging innate and adaptive immunity in atopic dermatitis. J Allergy Clin Immunol 2010;125:50–9.

10. Chinthrajah RS, Hernandez JD, Boyd SD, et al. Molecular and cellular mechanisms of food allergy and food tolerance. J Allergy Clin Immunol 2016;137(4):984–97.

11. Du Toit G, Roberts G, Sayre PH, et al. Identifying infants at high risk of peanut allergy: the Learning Early About Peanut Allergy (LEAP) screening study. J Allergy Clin Immunol 2013;131:135–43.

12. Wennergren G. What if it is the other way around? Early introduction of peanut and fish seems to be better than avoidance. Acta Paediatr 2009;98(7):1085–7.

13. Pape KA, Khoruts A, Mondino A, et al. Inflammatory cytokines enhance the in vivo clonal expansion and differentiation of antigen-activated CD4. J Immunol 1997;159:591–8.

14. Paul WE, Zhu J. How are T(H)2-type immune responses initiated and amplified? Nat Rev Immunol 2010;10:225–35.

15. Hardman CS, Chen YL, Salimi M, et al. CD1a presentation of endogenous antigens by group 2 innate lymphoid cells. Sci Immunol 2017;2(18) [pii: eaan5918].

16. Deckers J, Hammad H, Hoste E. Langerhans cells: sensing the environment in health and disease. Front Immunol 2018;9:93.

17. Palmer CN, Irvine AD, Terron-Kwiatkowski A, et al. Common loss-of-function variants of the epidermal barrier protein filaggrin are a major predisposing factor for atopic dermatitis. Nat Genet 2006;38:441–6.

18. Bin L, Leung DY. Genetic and epigenetic studies of atopic dermatitis. Allergy Asthma Clin Immunol 2016;12:52.

19. Ellenbogen Y, Jiménez-Saiz R, Spill P, et al. The initiation of Th2 immunity towards food allergens. Int J Mol Sci 2018;19(5) [pii:E1447].

20. Wu H, Deng Y, Zhao M, et al. Molecular control of follicular helper T cell development and differentiation. Front Immunol 2018;9:2470.

21. Redlich CA. Skin exposure and asthma: is there a connection? Proc Am Thorac Soc 2010;7(2):134–7.

22. Simpson EL, Chalmers JR, Hanifin JM, et al. Emollient enhancement of the skin barrier from birth offers effective atopic dermatitis prevention. J Allergy Clin Immunol 2014;134(4):818–23.

23. Horimukai K, Morita K, Narita M, et al. Application of moisturizer to neonates prevents development of atopic dermatitis. J Allergy Clin Immunol 2014;134(4):824–30.

24. Chieosilapatham P, Ogawa H, Niyonsaba F. Current insights into the role of human β-defensins in atopic dermatitis. Clin Exp Immunol 2017;190(2):155–66.

25. Bjerre RD, Bandier J, Skov L, et al. The role of the skin microbiome in atopic dermatitis: a systematic review. Br J Dermatol 2017;177(5):1272–8.

26. Hammond M, et al. The Skin Microbiome in Atopic Dermatitis: Interactions Between Bacteria and Fungi. Presented at the British Society for Investigative Dermatology Annual Meeting, Bradford, UK: April 3, 2019.

27. Reichert B, Salem I, Schrom K, et al. Unpublished data 2018.

28. Hurwitz RM, Rivera HP, Guin JD. Black-spot poison ivy dermatitis. An acute irritant contact dermatitis superimposed upon an allergic contact dermatitis. Am J Dermatopathol 1984;6(4):319–22.

29. Kelterer D, Bauer A, Elsner P. Spill-induced sensitization to isophoronediamine. Contact Dermatitis 2000;43(2):110.

30. Puza CJ, Atwater AR. Positive patch test reaction in a patient taking dupilumab. Dermatitis 2018;29(2):89.

31. Onoue A, Kabashima K, Kobayashi M, et al. Induction of eosinophil- and Th2-attracting epidermal chemokines and cutaneous late-phase reaction in tape-stripped skin. Exp Dermatol 2009;18(12):1036–43.

32. Scheman A, Patel KR, Roszko K, et al. American Contact Dermatitis Society Contact Allergy Management Program: Relative Prevalence of Contact Allergens from 2018 in North America. Dermatitis 2019;30(2):87–105.

33. Erfurt-Berge C, Geier J, Mahler V. The current spectrum of contact sensitization in patients with chronic leg ulcers or stasis dermatitis - new data from the Information Network of Departments of Dermatology (IVDK). Contact Dermatitis 2017;77(3):151–8.

34. Barbaud A, Poreaux C, Penven E, et al. Occupational protein contact dermatitis. Eur J Dermatol 2015;25(6):527–34.

35. Fisher AA. The paraben paradox. Cutis 1973;1:830.
36. Paulsen E, Christensen LP, Andersen KE. Tomato contact dermatitis. Contact Dermatitis 2012;67(6): 321–7.
37. Hjorth N, Roed-Petersen J. Occupational protein contact dermatitis in food handlers. Contact Dermatitis 1976;2(1):28–42.
38. Glatz M, Bosshard P, Schmid-Grendelmeier P. The role of fungi in atopic dermatitis. Immunol Allergy Clin North Am 2017;37(1):63–74.
39. Jinnestål CL, Belfrage E, Bäck O, et al. Skin barrier impairment correlates with cutaneous Staphylococcus aureus colonization and sensitization to skin-associated microbial antigens in adult patients with atopic dermatitis. Int J Dermatol 2014;53(1):27–33.
40. Niiyama S, TamauchiH, Amoh Y, et al. Th2 immune response plays a critical role in the development of nickel-induced allergic contact dermatitis. Int Arch Allergy Immunol 2010;153(3):303–14.
41. Dhingra N, Shemer A, Correa da Rosa J, et al. Molecular profiling of contact dermatitis skin identifies allergen-dependent differences in immune response. J Allergy Clin Immunol 2014;134(2): 362–72.
42. Machler BC, Sung CT, Darwin E, et al. Dupilumab use in allergic contact dermatitis. J Am Acad Dermatol 2019;80(1):280–1.
43. Garrido-Ríos AA, Martínez-Morán C, Borbujo J. Eccema dishidrótico secundario a la infusión de inmunoglobulinas intravenosas: presentación de 2 casos. Actas Dermosifiliogr 2016;107:431–3.
44. Jiménez-Saiz R, Ellenbogen Y, Koenig JFE, et al. IgG1(+) B-cell immunity predates IgE responses in epicutaneous sensitization to foods. Allergy 2019; 74(1):165–75.
45. Sánchez-Pérez J, Diez MB, Pérez AA, et al. Allergic and systemic contact dermatitis to methylparaben. Contact Dermatitis 2006;54(2):117–8.
46. Vandersall A, Katta R. Eyelid dermatitis as a manifestation of systemic contact dermatitis to cinnamon. Dermatitis 2015;26(4):189.
47. Rundle CW, Jacob SE, Machler BC. Contact dermatitis to carmine. Dermatitis 2018;29(5):244–9.
48. Pereira F, Hatia M, Cardoso J. Systemic contact dermatitis from diallyl disulfide. Contact Dermatitis 2002;46(2):124.
49. Burden AD, Wilkinson SM, Beck MH, et al. Garlic-induced systemic contact dermatitis. Contact Dermatitis 1994;46:299–315.
50. Rademaker M, Yung A. Contact dermatitis to Asparagus officinalis. Australas J Dermatol 2000;41(4): 262–3.
51. Scott JF, Conic RRZ, Kim I, et al. Atopy and sensitization to allergens known to cause systemic contact dermatitis. Dermatitis 2019;30(1):62–6.
52. Jensen CS, Lisby S, Larsen JK, et al. Characterization of lymphocyte subpopulations and cytokine profiles in peripheral blood of nickel-sensitive individuals with systemic contact dermatitis after oral nickel exposure. Contact Dermatitis 2004; 50(1):31–8.
53. Raison-Peyron N, Meynadier JM, Meynadier J. Sorbic acid: an unusual cause of systemic contact dermatitis in an infant. Contact Dermatitis 2000;43: 247.
54. Lowther A, McCormick T, Nedorost S. Systemic contact dermatitis from propylene glycol. Dermatitis 2008;19(2):105–8.
55. Jacob SE, Sung CT, Machler BC. Dupilumab for systemic allergy syndrome with dermatitis. Dermatitis 2019;30(2):164–7.
56. Stout M, Silverberg JI. Variable impact of dupilumab on patch testing results and allergic contact dermatitis in adults with atopic dermatitis. J Am Acad Dermatol 2019;81(1):157–62.

American Contact Dermatitis Society Allergens of the Year 2000 to 2020

Michelle Militello, MS[a,1], Sophia Hu, BA[b,2], Melissa Laughter, PhD[a,2], Cory A. Dunnick, MD[c,d,*]

KEYWORDS

- Allergic contact dermatitis • Patch testing • American Contact Dermatitis Society • Allergen
- Acrylates Dyes Medications • Metals • Rubber Accelerators Preservatives • Surfactants

KEY POINTS

- Allergic contact dermatitis is a prevalent delayed, type IV, hypersensitivity skin reaction to external stimuli.
- Patterns of dermatitis depend on allergen exposure and patch testing is the gold standard to identify causal agents.
- The American Contact Dermatitis Society identifies an "Allergen of the Year" in order to highlight interesting facts about particular allergens, which may range from showing increasing prevalence of disease, to documenting low levels of relevant allergic reactions.
- Categories of allergens reviewed include adhesives, dyes, medications, metals, preservatives, rubber accelerators, surfactants, and other skin care product ingredients.

INTRODUCTION

Allergic contact dermatitis (ACD) is a widespread skin condition affecting more than 14 million Americans each year.[1] ACD is a T cell–mediated, delayed type IV hypersensitivity reaction to exogenous agents and external stimuli.[2] Patterns of ACD depend on allergen exposures, and any body part that comes into contact with the allergen may develop an inflammatory reaction.[3] ACD may also occur secondary to treatment of an underlying disease, as seen in patients who develop allergies to topical corticosteroids and antibacterial creams.

A thorough medical history and epicutaneous patch testing can lead to identification of the responsible allergens, implementation of an avoidance regimen, and better patient outcomes.[3] With appropriate allergen avoidance, ACD may resolve and further episodes of dermatitis may be prevented, leading to significantly improved quality of life and decreased health care costs.[1]

The Allergen of the Year is an annual award approved by the American Contact Dermatitis Society (ACDS) to draw attention to common and often under-recognized agents causing significant ACD as well as those that do not cause

Funding sources: None.
[a] Rocky Vista University, College of Osteopathic Medicine, Parker, CO, USA; [b] University of Colorado School of Medicine, Aurora, CO, USA; [c] Department of Dermatology, University of Colorado, Anschutz Medical Campus, Aurora, CO, USA; [d] Rocky Mountain Regional Veterans Affairs Medical Center, Aurora, CO, USA
[1] present address: 8401 S Chambers Rd, Parker, CO 80134, USA
[2] present address: 12705 East Montview Avenue Suite 100 Aurora, CO, 8004, USA
* Corresponding author. 1665 Aurora Court, MS F703, Aurora, CO 80045.
E-mail address: cory.dunnick@cuanschutz.edu

Dermatol Clin 38 (2020) 309–320
https://doi.org/10.1016/j.det.2020.02.011
0733-8635/20/Published by Elsevier Inc.

derm.theclinics.com

significant allergy.[3] The awards have played a key role from both an academic standpoint and in generating increased public awareness. This article characterizes the ACDS Allergens of the Year from years 2000 to 2020 and discusses their significance from a clinical perspective (**Table 1**).

METHODS

The list of top contact allergens of the year was compiled from years 2000 to 2020 using the ACDS database. Categories of allergens included metals, preservatives, medications, skin care products, surfactants, and clothing-associated allergens. A comprehensive review of the literature of each ingredient was conducted on PubMed (US National Library of Medicine). Individual search terms specific to the names of the ingredients and associated terms were input into the advanced search tool to identify all articles discussing the relationship between the active ingredients and contact allergic dermatitis. Both in vitro and in vivo studies with publication dates up to 2019 were included. Non–English-language articles were excluded. A total of 62 references were used for this study.

DYES
Disperse Blue Dyes

The earliest written record of the use of natural dyes was found in China, dated 2600 BC. These initial records illustrate techniques for dyeing silk using various dyes derived from plants. In 1856, William H. Perkin accidentally created the first synthetic dye while attempting to create a possible cure for malaria.[4] Now, more than 1200 dye pigments are used in the textile industry. Dyes may be classified by their chemical structure or they may also be grouped within their chemical class based on their application.

Disperse dyes are classified by their application, based on the procedure involved in applying the dye to fabric. Disperse dyes are primarily used to color polyester, acetate fibers, and nylon fibers; they are particularly used in the dyeing of garments and stockings.[5] Because of their partial water solubility, and subsequent leaching out of fabrics and onto the skin, disperse dyes are the most common dye sensitizers. Disperse blue 124 and 106 are the most routinely positive dye sensitizers. In 2 studies published in 2000, 18% and 40% of the patients suspected of having a textile ACD had positive patch tests to textile dyes, with disperse blue dyes being the most prevalent. This finding led to disperse blue dyes being named the first

---

Table 1
"Allergens of the Year" 2000 to 2020

Adhesives and Rubber Accelerators	Dyes
Acrylates 2012	Disperse blue 2000
Mixed dialkyl thioureas 2009	p-Phenylenediamine 2006
Isobornyl acrylate 2020	—
—	*Metals*
Medications	Cobalt 2016
Bacitracin 2003	Gold 2001
Neomycin 2010	Nickel 2008
Glucocorticoids 2005	—
—	*Surfactants*
Preservatives	Alkyl glucosides 2017
Formaldehyde 2015	Cocamidopropyl betaine 2004
Methylisothiazolinone Methylchloroisothiazolinone 2013	—
Parabens 2019	*Other Skin Care Product Ingredients*
Thimerosal 2002	Benzophenones 2014
Dimethyl fumarate 2011	Fragrance 2007
—	Propylene glycol 2018

Allergen (Year Recognized)

Contact Allergen of the Year in 2000. The classic presentation of dye dermatitis is in the distribution of contact with the responsible garment. In addition, areas of increased friction, including the axillae, thighs, buttocks, and popliteal fossa, tend to be most often affected.[5]

Paraphenylenediamine

Paraphenylenediamine (PPD) is an ingredient widely used in hair dye, as well as in textiles, furs, and more recently henna. PPD was first introduced in 1880s and has since been the leading permanent hair-coloring agent. Most exposure to PPD occurs through hair color among consumers as well as among hairdressers. PPD is a strong sensitizer and is allergenic before it is oxidized; it is no longer allergenic after completing the hair dye process. Not surprisingly, allergy to PPD usually presents as dermatitis of the face near the hairline and neck, and may also involve the eyelids (**Fig. 1**). In addition to reactions related to hair coloring, PPD is an azo dye, similar in structure to the disperse dyes used to dye textiles and fur, and can therefore be a cause of textile or clothing dye dermatitis. Recently, reports of reactions to henna have also been reported. Henna is a greenish natural powder obtained from the flowers and dry leaves of the *Lawsonia alba* plant. When henna is used on its

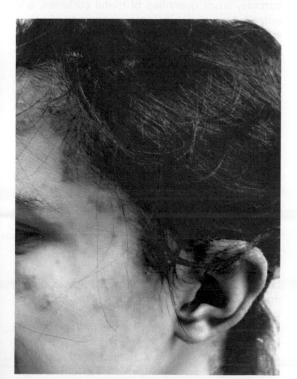

Fig. 1. A severe allergic reaction to hair dye in a patient found to be allergic to paraphenylenediamine.

own, it stains the skin a reddish brown; this is called red henna. In contrast, black henna is the combination of red henna with PPD and is used in order to darken the henna. When used by itself, henna has a very low allergenicity; however, when used with PPD, henna has been reported to cause significant ACD.[6] In most such cases, PPD has been determined as the offending agent.[7]

Although PPD has been around for more than a century, numerous changes have occurred in the clinical aspects of dealing with allergy to this antigen. These changes include the appreciation of new patterns of exposure that have led to increased sensitization potential, as seen in PPD-tainted henna tattoos, and increased usage as means to stave off the appearance of aging. For this reason, in 2006 PPD was named the ACDS Allergen of the Year.[7]

MEDICATIONS
Bacitracin

Bacitracin is an inexpensive and readily available topical antibiotic commonly used for the treatment and prophylaxis of local infections, burn injuries, and superficial wounds. Discovered in 1943, bacitracin gets its antimicrobial properties by blocking bacterial cell wall and peptidoglycan synthesis.[8] Bacitracin comes in many vehicles, including ointment, powders, and aerosols. Furthermore, bacitracin is commonly found in combination with other topical antibiotics sold over the counter, including triple antibiotic ointment with neomycin and polymyxin B (eg, Neosporin; Johnson & Johnson).[9] Although considered an effective, safe, and harmless medication, bacitracin is a sensitizer and can cause not only ACD but also urticarial reactions and near-fatal anaphylaxis. Data from the North American Contact Dermatitis Group (NACDG) identified bacitracin as the ninth most common allergen in 1998 to 2000, causing 9.2% of positive reactions. Bacitracin's wide clinical use for several years may have been responsible for its exposure and sensitization in the population at large.[10] For this reason, bacitracin was named Allergen of the Year in 2003.

Neomycin

Neomycin is a commonly used antibiotic complex composed of structurally similar aminoglycosides (neomycin A, B, and C). It is produced by the growth of *Streptomyces fradiae* and works by binding to bacterial ribosomal RNA, leading to inhibition of protein synthesis.[8] Neomycin is indicated for the prophylaxis and treatment of superficial infections in wounds and burns. Neomycin is commonly available as a 20% neomycin sulfate solution in various delivery vehicles or combined with other topical antimicrobials.[8]

Neomycin is generally considered safe and effective and can be purchased over the counter; however, ACD is a well-known side effect of topically applied neomycin.[11] Contact allergy to neomycin must be distinguished from infection, especially when used postoperatively (**Fig. 2**). Neomycin contact sensitization peaked at 13.1% in 1996 to 1998 according to review of NACDG data, with allergy prevalence of 7% in 2015 to 2016 NACDG data, and is still the seventh most commonly positive patch-test ingredient.[12] Neomycin is known to cross react with most other aminoglycoside antibiotics, including tobramycin, gentamycin, streptomycin, and amikacin, and, in order to highlight these facts, neomycin was named ACDS Allergen of the Year in 2010.

Glucocorticoids

Although topical corticosteroids (CSs) are the mainstay of treatment of ACD, they can also sometimes cause ACD themselves. The first reported case of ACD to corticosteroids was

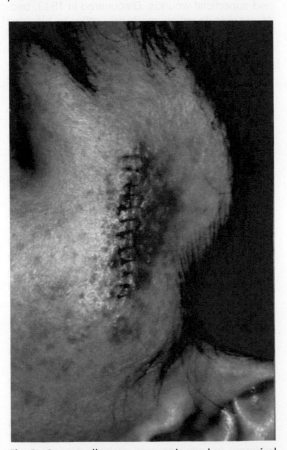

Fig. 2. Contact allergy to neomycin used on a surgical wound.

reported in the 1950s.[13] Importantly, the ACD reaction to CS is not thought to be caused by the CS but instead by the breakdown products formed during the degradation of the product. The byproduct produced during CS degradation is a CS-glyoxal protein complex that may serve as a hapten capable of producing an allergic reaction.[14] The prevalence of ACD to CS ranges from 0.2% to 0.5%.[15] In 2000, 1 study conducted at the Mayo Clinic showed that, of 1188 patients tested, 3% to 6% had a reaction to at least 1 class of topical steroid. Furthermore, each CS has a risk of cross reacting with another CS within its respective class.[16] One study examining 41 patients showed cross reactivities of ACD ranging from 20% to 80% depending on the classes of CS compared.[17] This cross reactivity between steroid allergies is likely caused by the structural similarity of the compounds within each respective class. For all of these reasons, CSs were named ACDS Allergen of the Year in 2005.

METALS
Cobalt

Cobalt is a shiny, magnetic, brittle metal contained in a variety of materials.[18] The hard metal is manufactured by a powder metallurgical process that combines 10% metallic cobalt with 90% tungsten carbide, small quantities of metal carbides, and polyethylene glycol.[19] Common sources of cobalt exposure include tools, magnets, orthopedic and medical devices, ceramics, cement, plastics, and leather. Cobalt allergy is less common than nickel, and cosensitization can occur because metals often contain both elements.[19,20] Cobalt is a strong skin sensitizer and the occurrence of localized contact dermatitis has been documented in hard metal workers.[19,21,22] In contrast, systemic contact dermatitis (SCD) is rarely caused by contact with hard metal powder. There has been only 1 report of occupational cobalt-induced SCD, in which a hard metal factory worker developed a generalized eczematous eruption with pruritus that resolved after the allergen was removed.[23]

Moreover, although exceedingly uncommon, there have also been reports of allergy to the cobalt contained within vitamin B_{12} (cyanocobalamin). Allergy to cyanocobalamin was found in 2 patients shown to be sensitive to cobalt to patch testing. One patient who was found to be allergic to cobalt ingested B12 tablets regularly and developed recurrent cheilitis. A patient who was found to be allergic to cobalt ingested B_{12} tablets regularly and developed recurrent cheilitis.[18] This same patient later developed stomatitis of the hard palate when her dentist inadvertently made her a denture out of a cobalt alloy. In addition, Fisher reported 1 cobalt-allergic patient that correlated with an allergic reaction to an injectable vitamin B_{12}. This patient had a positive patch test to cobalt chloride and vitamin B_{12}.[4] The increase in the number of sources of cobalt exposure as well as the development of the cobalt spot test to identify cobalt-containing products led cobalt to be named 2016 Allergen of the Year.

Gold

Gold is an easily malleable noble metal that is resistant to corrosion, making it useful in medicine and dentistry as well as other industries.[24] It is frequently used in jewelry, dental crowns, medical implants, and cosmetics. Gold is the second most frequent allergen after nickel among patients with piercings.[25,26] Although metallic gold is widely nonsensitizing, gold salts such as gold sodium thiosulfate may elicit allergic reactions identified by positive patch tests.[27] Interpretation of gold reactions in patch testing is problematic, because gold may be associated with significantly delayed and persistent reactions that are often irrelevant.[24] Gold contact dermatitis is usually seen in occupational exposures, and areas of skin where makeup and jewelry are contacted.[24] Common areas of involvement include the eyelids, ears, hands, and neck and may take the form of a chronic papular eruption. Many studies have also substantiated the role of gold exposure in causing SCD, and oral gold may lead to the development of lichen planus–like eruptions (**Fig. 3**).[24] Intramuscular

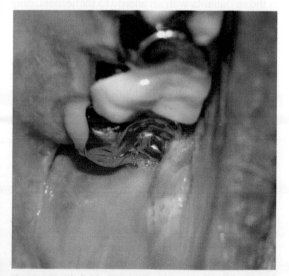

Fig. 3. Oral lichen planus–like eruption on the buccal mucosa in a patient allergic to gold in these dental prostheses.

gold sodium thiomalate therapy for rheumatoid arthritis, and gold-containing supplements, have been reported to induce SCD.[28–30] Overall, recognition of gold as a possible cause of ACD, but with many irrelevant positive patch-test results, led it to be designated as the 2001 Allergen of the Year.

Nickel

Nickel is a natural element and transition metal found ubiquitously in the environment.[19] It makes up 3% of the earth's composition and is widely used in the manufacturing of metal alloys.[31,32] Common sources of nickel exposure include zippers, safety pins, doorknobs, keys, scissors, eyelash curlers, belt buckles, metal eyeglass frames, multivitamins, jewelry, mobile phones, and nickel-plated objects.[3] According to the NACDG patch-test results from 2015 to 2016, nickel remained the most prevalent allergen, with 17.5% positivity in those who are patch tested worldwide.[12] According to recent studies, women have a 4-fold higher relative risk of developing contact dermatitis to nickel compared with men.[31] Furthermore, a positive correlation was found between filaggrin mutations, atopic dermatitis, and contact sensitization to nickel.[33] Sensitized individuals usually experience a localized cutaneous eruption with erythema, vesicle formation, desquamation, and pruritus.[19] Dermatitis is commonly localized to the earlobes, neck, wrists, and periumbilical areas because of contact with jewelry or belt buckles. The metal does not usually cause SCD, because it is usually manufactured into nickel-steel alloys or stainless steel.[34] However, nickel may be released from its innocuous form when exposed to organic acids, especially when cooked at high temperatures.[35] Thus, SCD can occur with dietary ingestion of nickel[19] and foods such as beans, chocolate, nuts, and oatmeal are especially high in nickel content. The utility of a low-nickel diet is controversial, but avoidance of cutaneous exposure to metal objects is recommended for nickel-sensitive individuals. The high prevalence of contact dermatitis to nickel, as well as the evidence that supports regulation to decrease nickel sensitization, led to its designation as 2008 ACDS Allergen of the Year.

PRESERVATIVES
Formaldehyde

Formaldehyde is a biocidal preservative used in both skin care products and within industry. Formaldehyde has been incorporated into a vast array of products, including nail polish, personal hygiene products, wrinkle-free clothing, Brazilian blowout treatments, plastics, textiles, and protective gloves. The use of formaldehyde has decreased over time because of its carcinogenic potential and sensitizing effects. Formaldehyde-releasing preservatives (FRPs) were subsequently developed with the idea that the amount of formaldehyde released would not be enough to cause a contact allergy. FRPs including quaternium-15, imidazolidinyl urea, diazolidinyl urea, DMDM hydantoin, and bronopol have replaced formaldehyde in personal care products, makeup, medications, and household cleaning products. Sources of FRPs include shampoos, body washes, hand soaps, lotions, baby wipes, mascara, disinfectants, fabric softeners, and topical wart remedies.[36]

Because of its incorporation in both cosmetics, fabrics, and industrial products, via FRPs, formaldehyde is not only an important cosmetic source of allergic dermatitis but it is also an important source of occupational dermatitis. In 2015, it was designated the ACDS Allergen of the Year.[37]

Methylisothiazolinone and Methylchloroisothiazolinone (Isothiazolinones)

The preservative pair, methylchloroisothiazolinone (MCI) with methylisothiazolinone (MI), was first introduced in 1980 in a 3:1 combination. MCI/MI offered a substitute for formaldehyde because of their lower rates of sensitization and less concern for toxicity. Soon after their introduction as preservatives, rates of contact allergy to MCI/MI increased to levels of up to 8%. In the early 2000s, MI alone was approved for use as a preservative for industrial and cosmetic products because it was thought to be a weaker sensitizer than MCI. MI alone was also determined to be a less effective biocide than the combination of MCI/MI, and therefore MI was approved for use in higher concentrations, which has led to the current epidemic of MCI/MI contact allergy. Notably, a positive reaction to MI can be missed if a patient is patch tested only to the combination of MCI/MI; therefore, testing to MI alone is necessary to screen for allergy to these preservatives.[38]

Exposure to MI can derive from both cosmetic and occupational sources. For example, MI was incorporated into moist toilet papers, prompting a wave of perianal dermatitis, and later into makeup remover wipes, leading to several cases of eyelid and facial dermatitis.[36] In addition, the first occupational exposure to MI was reported in 2004, in which the ACD came from exposure to wallpaper glue.[38] There are other hidden sources of MI, including acrylic paint and homemade slime, which is popular with children. In 2013, MI was named the ACDS Allergen of the Year.

Parabens

For more than 70 years, parabens have been extensively used as preservatives in cosmetics, food, and pharmaceuticals. Parabens have become a popular choice among the preservatives because of their lack of taste and odor, and relatively neutral pH. According to the Contact Allergen Management Program (CAMP) data, of the 4612 products listed, parabens were present in 19% of them. Within this family, methylparaben, ethylparaben, propylparaben, and butylparaben are the most commonly used, both independently and with other preservatives. Without preservation, cosmetic products, food, and pharmaceuticals rapidly become contaminated with mold, fungi, and bacteria, leading to spoilage and increased risks for infection, thus necessitating the need for preservatives such as parabens.[39]

Despite misguided apprehension about parabens being harmful, the US Food and Drug Administration have classified parabens as generally safe. They remain one of the least allergenic preservatives available and are rarely problematic as contact allergens. For this reason, parabens were designated the ACDS Nonallergen of the Year in 2019.[39]

Thimerosal

Thimerosal is a mercury-containing compound that has been used as an antiseptic and preservative in several vaccines, cosmetic products, and topical drugs.[40] According to the NACDG, from 1996 to 1998, thimerosal was the fifth most common allergen in 10.9% of 4087 patients. However, in those patients with an allergy to thimerosal, only 16.8% of them were considered to have a thimerosal allergy relevant to their dermatitis.[41] Of note, the prevalence of thimerosal sensitization was presumed to be induced by vaccinations, because thimerosal was used as a preservative in vaccines up until 1999.[42] Routine testing to thimerosal is no longer recommended and thus thimerosal was the first to be recognized as a Nonallergen of the Year in 2002 given its frequently positive, but often irrelevant, reactions on patch testing.

Dimethyl Fumarate

Dimethyl fumarate (DMF) is a fumaric acid ester that has been used in the treatment of psoriasis for more than 20 years and is also a preservative in desiccant sachets found in the packaging of furniture and shoes.[43,44] DMF has been shown to be an effective mold inhibitor and is therefore used in the overseas transportation of furniture and shoes to prevent mold formation.

Beginning in 2007, an epidemic of ACD occurred in Europe. A relapsing dermatitis present on the backs and buttocks was reported in several Finnish patients. One of the patients tested positive to a textile fabric from a Chinese reclining chair. Subsequently, nearly 100 cases of dermatitis related to reclining chairs manufactured in China were reported in Finland. The inciting allergen was later identified as DMF.

Owing to the random distribution of the DMF-containing sachets inside Chinese chairs, the localization of the dermatitis depends on where the patient has contact with the fabric. However, commonly affected areas include the trunk, limbs, buttocks, and face. Blistering and lichenoid reactions can be seen as well as contact urticaria.[37] In 2009, the European Commission banned importation of products containing greater than the maximum allowable amount of DMF because of the increasing incidence of allergic reactions to furniture and footwear. Even though DMF is still used overseas, there have been no case reports of allergy in patients in North America. In 2011, DMF was chosen as the Allergen of the Year to show the rapid identification and regulation of a previously unrecognized cause of ACD.

SURFACTANTS
Alkyl Glucosides

Alkyl glucosides are plant-derived biodegradable surfactants that have been around for more than 4 decades. Although they are not necessarily new surfactants, they were recently rediscovered because of their eco-friendly character, and their use has been steadily increasing. For example, they are classically included in a variety of household products, including cosmetics, skin care items, hair dyes, cleansers, and tanning formulations.[45] In addition, the leave-on cosmetic products most frequently associated with glucoside-associated ACD include sunscreens and facial moisturizers. ACD to alkyl glucosides is most often caused by the lauryl and decyl glucoside subtypes and is more common in individuals with a history of atopy.[46] As a result of increased reports of sensitivity to decyl glucoside, it was introduced to the NACDG standard patch testing series in 2009. The rate of positive patch-test reactions to decyl glucoside has increased from 1.3% in 2014 to 2.2% in 2016.[47] Moreover, although alkyl glucosides are generally considered to be mild in terms of their ability to produce allergy, reports of contact dermatitis to this family of molecules have been increasingly common, leading it to be named the ACDS Allergen of the Year for 2017.

Cocamidopropyl Betaine

Cocamidopropyl betaine is an amphoteric synthetic detergent that has been steadily increasing in the use of cosmetics and personal hygiene products, including shampoos, contact lens, toothpaste, detergents, makeup removers, bath gels, cleansers, liquid soaps, antiseptics, and gynecologic and anal hygiene products. Of the 19,000 cosmetic products registered in 1980, 0.25% of them contained cocamidopropyl betaine. By 2005, 5.6% of 22,016 products listed contained cocamidopropyl betaine, indicating a significant increase in prevalence. Of note, cocamidopropyl betaine is most well known for its use in baby and gentle shampoos because it is less irritating and mild compared with other surfactants, including sodium lauryl sulfate. However, although less irritating, cocamidopropyl betaine is more likely to cause allergic sensitization (**Fig. 4**).[4]

Cocamidopropyl betaine allergy typically presents as eyelid, facial, scalp, and/or neck dermatitis. This pattern is likely explained by frequent exposure to personal cleansing products and/or the enhanced proclivity of these areas to develop allergic contact dermatitis.[4] The prevalence of contact sensitization to cocamidopropyl betaine continues to increase, and, for that reason, it was designated the ACDS Allergen of the Year for 2004.[4]

OTHER SKIN CARE PRODUCT INGREDIENTS
Benzophenone

Benzophenone is added to personal care products and commercial solutions in order to protect against the damaging effects of ultraviolet light. Initially, benzophenones were used as

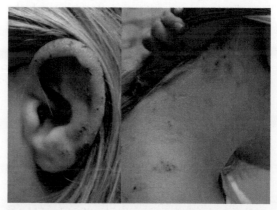

Fig. 4. ACD to cocamidopropyl betaine showing a classic pattern of rash found with allergy to ingredients in shampoo.

preservatives in industrial products such as paints, varnishes, and plastics to extend shelf life and reduce photodegradation. By the 1950s, they were introduced as sunscreens as effective absorbers of both ultraviolet A and B.[48] They are now present in topical sunscreens as well as other cosmetics, including moisturizers, hair sprays, perfumes, shampoos, detergent bars, and nail polish. Cosmetics account for most exposures to these allergens; however, reactions secondary to industrial exposures also exist.

There are 3 benzophenones approved for use in sunscreens in the United States: benzophenone-3, benzophenone-4, and benzophenone-8. The first documented case of ACD to benzophenone-3 (oxybenzone) was in 1972.[49] Since then, benzophenones have been documented to cause numerous adverse cutaneous reactions, including contact and photocontact dermatitis, contact and photocontact urticaria, and anaphylaxis. Oxybenzone is not only the most common benzophenone to cause positive patch-test reactions but also the most common ultraviolet filter, overall, to cause allergy. As a group, benzophenones were named the ACDS Allergen of the Year for 2014 in order to raise awareness of both allergy and photoallergy to these ubiquitous agents.[50]

Fragrance

Fragrances are a group of naturally derived and synthetic chemicals known for their odor-enhancing or odor-blending properties. Because of their unique properties, they are often incorporated into food, industrial, cosmetic, and hygienic products. There are more than 2800 fragrance ingredients listed in the database of the Research Institute for Fragrance Materials Inc, and, of those, at least 100 are known allergens.[51] In addition, new fragrance allergens can also be hidden ingredients on cosmetic and cleaning products, even in those that are marketed as fragrance free.[36]

In the late 1970s Dr Walter Larson developed fragrance mix I (FM I) to be used as an important screening marker for contact allergies to fragrances. FM I consists of 8 fragrance chemicals: eugenol, isoeugenol, cinnamaldehyde, hydroxycitronellal, geraniol, cinnamyl alcohol, and amyl cinnamal. and *Evernia prunastri* (oakmoss). Although these 8 chemicals continue to be relevant fragrance allergens, a need for an expanded fragrance mix was acknowledged in the 1990s, when research suggested that 15% of pertinent perfume allergies were not identified by FM I.[52] Fragrance mix II was then introduced in 2005, which included the chemicals, Lyral, citral,

citronellol, farnesol, coumarin, and hexyl-cinnamic aldehyde. Fragrance mix II was able to identify additional patients with fragrance sensitivities missed by FM I.[36] Fragrances are complex substances and any 1 perfume may contain hundreds of different chemicals. Attempting to pinpoint specific fragrance allergens has challenged patch testing for years, and it will continue to do so as new fragrance allergies continue to emerge. Recently, using essential oils as home remedies has been become popular. However, the strong concentrations of fragrances in essential oils can lead to contact sensitization and contact allergy (**Fig. 5**). In order to highlight its prevalence as a contact allergen, it was chosen as the 2007 Allergen of the Year.[51]

Propylene Glycol

Propylene glycol is a synthetic alcohol with emollient, solvent, antimicrobial, and emulsifying properties. It is commonly used in cosmetics, personal hygiene products, medications (including topical corticosteroids), food products, and recently electronic cigarettes.[53] The use of propylene glycol has significantly increased since its introduction in the 1930s, and it is now present in more than 37% of the 4674 products logged in the ACDS 2016 CAMP database.

Of note, patch testing for propylene glycol and its relevance as a contact allergen is debated; this is because of its ability to act as a weak

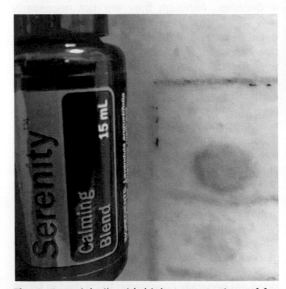

Fig. 5. Essential oils with high concentrations of fragrances can lead to contact sensitization, as seen with this positive patch-test reaction to a blend containing lavender, ylang ylang, marjoram, Roman chamomile, Hawaiian sandalwood, and vanilla.

sensitizer and an irritant. Because of this, the results of a positive patch test to propylene glycol may be difficult. Nevertheless, many patients manifest some form of sensitivity and, despite the controversy of propylene glycol as an irritant versus an allergic reactant, any reaction is pertinent to the patients whose skin is compromised. Allergic and irritant contact dermatitis as well as systemic cutaneous reactions to propylene glycol have been documented, which therefore led this allergen to be named the ACDS Allergen of the Year for 2018.[54]

ADHESIVES AND RUBBER ACCELERATORS
Acrylates

Acrylates are plastic constituents that are formed by the polymerization of monomers derived from acrylic or methacrylic acid. The monomeric building blocks, acrylates, and to a lesser extent methacrylates are not only strong irritants but are also notorious allergens. Acrylates are used widely in dental composite resins, printing inks, artificial nails, as well as medical devices such as contact lenses and hearing aids.

Since the 1950s, there have been numerous case reports documenting the contact dermatitis caused by these plastic constituents. For instance, methyl methacrylate (MMA), which was previously used in artificial nails, caused severe periungual dermatitis, often accompanied by nail destruction and persistent paresthesia (**Fig. 6**).[55] For this reason, MMA was banned for use in artificial nails by the Food and Drug Administration in 1974. However, acrylate alternatives have since replaced this allergen and seem to be just as sensitizing as MMA. Because of this, acrylates were named the ACDS Allergen of the Year for 2012.[55]

Mixed Dialkyl Thiourea

Dialkyl thiourea is an organic compound commonly found in rubber (neoprene in particular), glues, textiles, insecticides, and in the photocopying and photographic industries as antioxidants and fixatives.[56] Of the various products containing dialkyl thiourea, many cases of ACD from neoprene have been reported, including cases caused by rubber orthopedic braces, prostheses, splints, athletic shoes, rubber masks, swim goggles, and wet suits (**Fig. 7**).[56]

Although thioureas have long been used as an industrial compound, the first cases of ACD were reported in the 1960s. Since then, the increased use and prevalence of dialkyl thioureas have led to their general acceptance as a cause of ACD.[57] The NACDG collected data on patch-tested patients using mixed dialkyl thioureas (MDTUs), which showed a positive patch-test reaction to MDTU in 0.7% to 1.3% of patients.[58] In a similar

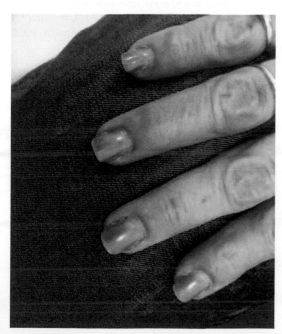

Fig. 6. ACD to acrylates in artificial nails.

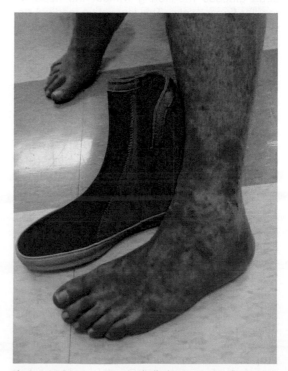

Fig. 7. ACD to mixed dialkyl thiourea found in neoprene shoes used for waterskiing.

study, the Mayo Clinic dermatology clinics reported that 2.4% of 1368 patients showed a positive patch-test reaction to various mixtures of dialkyl thiourea compounds.[59] In a larger, more recent retrospective analysis, 1% of 21,898 patients that were patch tested from 1994 to 2004 showed a positive reaction to MDTU, with 76.9% of these reactions being currently relevant and 17.1% being occupationally relevant.[58] For these reasons, dialkyl thiourea was designated Contact Allergen of the Year in 2009.

Isobornyl Acrylate

Isobornyl acrylate (IOBA) is a photopolymerizable monomer that has been used in industrial products such as ultraviolet-cured ink or adhesives. As a group, acrylates are well-known allergens in patients exposed to them in various settings: artificial nails, adhesives, dental composite fillings, dentures, hearing aids, and personal hygiene pads, to name a few.[60] IOBA has been highlighted as a significant allergen in order to bring attention to its role as an allergen in a new source: glucose monitoring systems and insulin pumps.

Glucose sensors such as FreeStyle Libre are ground-breaking medical devices developed for patients with diabetes as a replacement for classic glucose meters in order to allow continuous glucose monitoring without the need for regular finger sticks. This innovative medical device is applied to the skin with adhesive for up to 14 days. There have been reports of documented allergy to IOBA in both glucose monitoring systems and insulin pumps since 1995.[61] If contact allergy is suspected, testing IOBA 0.1% in petrolatum is recommended because IOBA rarely cross reacts with other acrylates on the standard screening panels. There are glucose monitoring systems that are free of IOBA, such as the Dexcom system, which may be safe alternatives for patients with diabetes.[62] IOBA was named as Allergen of the Year for 2020 to increase awareness of the medical exposures to IOBA and to highlight that routine screening with other acrylates may be insufficient to screen for this allergy.

SUMMARY

ACD remains one of the leading causes of skin disease and can significantly affect patients' quality of life. It is imperative that dermatologists accurately identify the offending allergen to properly treat this condition and stop the progression of symptoms. For this reason, it is important that dermatologists be aware of the most common allergens present in commonly used skincare products, medications, clothing, and so forth. It is hoped that the knowledge provided in this article will improve understanding of the selection of the Allergens of the Year as well as help clinicians in their identification and treatment of ACD.

CONFLICTS OF INTEREST

None declared.

REFERENCES

1. Bickers DR, Lim HW, Margolis D, et al. The burden of skin diseases: 2004 a joint project of the American Academy of Dermatology Association and the Society for Investigative Dermatology. J Am Acad Dermatol 2006;55(3):490–500.
2. Schalock P. Common allergens in allergic contact dermatitis. Waltham, MA: UpToDate; 2019.
3. Dermatologist T. Review ACDS' Allergen of the Year 2000-2015. https://www.the-dermatologist.com/content/review-acds'-allergen-od-year-2000-2015. Accessed August 28, 2019.
4. Jacob SE, Atnini S. Cocamidopropyl betaine. Dermatitis 2008. https://doi.org/10.2310/6620.2008.06043.
5. Jacob SE, Ramirez CC. Focus on 2000 allergen of the year: textile dyes. Skin and Aging 2007;15(1): 28–34.
6. De Groot AC. Side-effects of henna and semi-permanent "black henna" tattoos: A full review. Contact Dermatitis 2013. https://doi.org/10.1111/cod.12074.
7. DeLeo VA. p-phenylenediamine. Dermatitis 2006. https://doi.org/10.2310/6620.2006.05054.
8. Porras-Luque JI. Topical antimicrobial agents in dermatology. Actas dermo-sifiliograficas 2007;98: 29–39.
9. Sugai T. Fisher's contact dermatitis. J Dermatol Sci 1996. https://doi.org/10.1016/s0923-1811(96)00511-7.
10. Sood A, Taylor JS. Bacitracin: allergen of the year. Am J Contact Dermat 2003. https://doi.org/10.2310/6620.2003.38621.
11. de Púdua CAM, Schnuch A, Lessmann H, et al. Contact allergy to neomycin sulfate: results of a multifactorial analysis. Pharmacoepidemiol Drug Saf 2005. https://doi.org/10.1002/pds.1117.
12. DeKoven JG, Warshaw EM, Zug KA, et al. North American Contact Dermatitis Group Patch Test Results: 2015-2016. Dermatitis 2018. https://doi.org/10.1097/DER.0000000000000417.
13. Burckhardt W. Contact eczema caused by hydrocortisone. Hautarzt 1959;10:42.
14. Wilkinson SM, Jones MF. Corticosteroid usage and binding to arginine: determinants of corticosteroid

hypersensitivity. Br J Dermatol 1996. https://doi.org/10.1111/j.1365-2133.1996.tb01151.x.

15. Baeck M, Marot L, Nicolas JF, et al. Allergic hypersensitivity to topical and systemic corticosteroids: a review. Allergy 2009. https://doi.org/10.1111/j.1398-9995.2009.02038.x.

16. Davis MDP, el-Azhary RA, Farmer SA. Results of patch testing to a corticosteroid series: a retrospective review of 1188 patients during 6 years at Mayo Clinic. J Am Acad Dermatol 2007. https://doi.org/10.1016/j.jaad.2006.11.012.

17. Gönül M, Gül Ü. Detection of contact hypersensitivity to corticosteroids in allergic contact dermatitis patients who do not respond to topical corticosteroids. Contact Dermatitis 2005. https://doi.org/10.1111/j.0105-1873.2005.00638.x.

18. Fowler JF Jr. Cobalt. Dermatitis 2016;27(1):3–8.

19. Yoshihisa Y, Shimizu T. Metal allergy and systemic contact dermatitis: an overview. Dermatol Res Pract 2012;2012:749561.

20. Shanon J. Pseudo-atopic dermatitis. Contact dermatitis due to chrome sensitivity simulating atopic dermatitis. Dermatologica 1965;131(3):176–90.

21. Schwartz L, Peck S, Kenneth B, et al. Allergic dermatitis due to metallic cobalt. J Allergy 1945;16(1):51–3.

22. Skog E. Skin affections caused by hard metal dust. Ind Med Surg 1963;32:266–8.

23. Asano Y, Makino T, Norisugi O, et al. Occupational cobalt induced systemic contact dermatitis. Eur J Dermatol 2009;19(2):166–7.

24. Chen JK, Lampel HP. Gold contact allergy: clues and controversies. Dermatitis 2015;26(2):69–77.

25. Nakada T, Iijima M, Nakayama H, et al. Role of ear piercing in metal allergic contact dermatitis. Contact Dermatitis 1997;36(5):233–6.

26. Sung CT, Machler BC, Jacob SE. Piercing metal contact allergy: nothing gold can stay. Dermatitis 2018;29(4):227–8.

27. Aberer W. Gold is precious-but a potent sensitizer? J Allergy Clin Immunol Pract 2019;7(1):294–5.

28. Moller H, Ohlsson K, Linder C, et al. Cytokines and acute phase reactants during flare-up of contact allergy to gold. Am J Contact Dermat 1998;9(1):15–22.

29. Moller H, Bjorkner B, Bruze M. Clinical reactions to systemic provocation with gold sodium thiomalate in patients with contact allergy to gold. Br J Dermatol 1996;135(3):423–7.

30. Moller H, Ohlsson K, Linder C, et al. The flare-up reactions after systemic provocation in contact allergy to nickel and gold. Contact Dermatitis 1999;40(4):200–4.

31. Lu LK, Warshaw EM, Dunnick CA. Prevention of nickel allergy: the case for regulation? Dermatol Clin 2009;27(2):155–61. vi-vii.

32. Barceloux DG. Nickel. J Toxicol Clin Toxicol 1999;37(2):239–58.

33. Novak N, Baurecht H, Schafer T, et al. Loss-of-function mutations in the filaggrin gene and allergic contact sensitization to nickel. J Invest Dermatol 2008;128(6):1430–5.

34. Rietschel RL, Fowler JF. Fisher's contact dermatitis. 6th edition. Hamilton (Canada): BC Deck Inc; 2008.

35. Kuligowski J, Halperin KM. Stainless steel cookware as a significant source of nickel, chromium, and iron. Arch Environ Contam Toxicol 1992;23(2):211–5.

36. Milam EC, Jacob SE, Cohen DE. Contact dermatitis in the patient with atopic dermatitis. J Allergy Clin Immunol Pract 2019. https://doi.org/10.1016/j.jaip.2018.11.003.

37. Bruze M, Zimerson E. Dimethyl fumarate. Dermatitis 2011. https://doi.org/10.2310/6620.2011.00002.

38. Castanedo-Tardana MP, Zug KA. Methylisothiazolinone. Dermatitis 2013. https://doi.org/10.1097/DER.0b013e31827edc73.

39. Fransway AF, Fransway PJ, Belsito DV, et al. Parabens. Dermatitis 2019. https://doi.org/10.1097/DER.0000000000000429.

40. Audicana MT, Munoz D, Dolores del Pozo M, et al. Allergic contact dermatitis from mercury antiseptics and derivatives: study protocol of tolerance to intramuscular injections of thimerosal. Am J Contact Dermat 2002;13(1):3–9.

41. Belsito DV. Thimerosal: contact (non)allergen of the year. Am J Contact Dermat 2002. https://doi.org/10.1053/ajcd.2002.31366.

42. Timeline: Thimerosal in Vaccines (1999-2010) Thimerosal | Concerns | Vaccine Safety | CDC. CDC. https://www.cdc.gov/vaccinesafety/concerns/thimerosal/timeline.html. Published 2015. Accessed December 20, 2019.

43. Blair HA. Dimethyl fumarate: a review in moderate to severe plaque psoriasis. Drugs 2018. https://doi.org/10.1007/s40265-017-0854-6.

44. Silvestre JF, Mercader P, Giménez-Arnau AM. Contact Dermatitis Due to Dimethyl Fumarate. Actas Dermosifiliogr 2010. https://doi.org/10.1016/s1578-2190(10)70619-3.

45. Alfalah M, Loranger C, Sasseville D. Alkyl Glucosides. Dermatitis 2017. https://doi.org/10.1097/DER.0000000000000234.

46. Loranger C, Alfalah M, Ferrier Le Bouedec MC, et al. Alkyl glucosides in contact dermatitis. Dermatitis 2017. https://doi.org/10.1097/DER.0000000000000240.

47. Milam EC, Cohen DE. Contact dermatitis: emerging trends. Dermatol Clin 2019. https://doi.org/10.1016/j.det.2018.07.005.

48. Knox JM, Guin J, Cockerell EG. Benzophenones; ultraviolet light absorbing agents. J Invest Dermatol 1957. https://doi.org/10.1038/jid.1957.119.

49. Ramsay DL, Cohen HJ, Baer RL. Allergic reaction to benzophenone: simultaneous occurrence of urticarial and contact sensitivities. Arch Dermatol 1972. https://doi.org/10.1001/archderm.1972.01620090076017.

50. Heurung AR, Raju SI, Warshaw EM. Benzophenones. Dermatitis 2014;25(1):3–10.

51. Storrs FJ, Belsito DV. Fragrance. Dermatitis 2007; 18(1):3–7.

52. De Groot AC, Van Der Kley AMJ, Bruynzeel DP, et al. Frequency of false-negative reactions to the fragrance mix. Contact Dermatitis 1993. https://doi.org/10.1111/j.1600-0536.1993.tb03373.x.

53. Lessmann H, Schnuch A, Geier J, et al. Skin-sensitizing and irritant properties of propylene glycol. Contact Dermatitis 2005. https://doi.org/10.1111/j.0105-1873.2005.00693.x.

54. McGowan MA, Scheman A, Jacob SE. Propylene glycol in contact dermatitis: a systematic review. Dermatitis 2018. https://doi.org/10.1097/DER.0000000000000307.

55. Sasseville D. Acrylates in contact dermatitis. Dermatitis 2012. https://doi.org/10.1097/DER.0b013e31823d1b81.

56. Anderson BE. Mixed dialkyl thioureas. Dermatitis 2009. https://doi.org/10.2310/6620.2008.08062.

57. Dooms-Goossens A, Chrispeels MT, De Veylder H, et al. Contact and photocontact sensitivity problems associated with thiourea and its derivatives: a review of the literature and case reports. Br J Dermatol 1987. https://doi.org/10.1111/j.1365-2133.1987.tb05881.x.

58. Warshaw EM, Cook JW, Belsito DV, et al. Positive patch-test reactions to mixed dialkyl thioureas: Cross-sectional data from the North American Contact Dermatitis Group, 1994 to 2004. Dermatitis 2008;19(4):190–201.

59. Comfere NI, Davis MDP, Fett DD. Patch-test reactions to thioureas are frequently relevant. Dermatitis 2005. https://doi.org/10.2310/6620.2005.05014.

60. Mowad CM. Glucose monitors: not as sweet as they seem. American Academy of Dermatology Association; 2019. Available at: https://www.aad.org/dw/dw-insights-and-inquiries/2019-archive/october/glucose-monitors-not-as-sweet-as-they-seem. Accessed December 30, 2019.

61. Raison-Peyron N, Mowitz M, Bonardel N, et al. Allergic contact dermatitis caused by isobornyl acrylate in OmniPod, an innovative tubeless insulin pump. Contact Dermatitis 2018. https://doi.org/10.1111/cod.12995.

62. Oppel E, Kamann S, Reichl FX, et al. The Dexcom glucose monitoring system—An isobornyl acrylate-free alternative for diabetic patients. Contact Dermatitis 2019. https://doi.org/10.1111/cod.13248.

Common Allergens and Considerations When Performing Pediatric Patch Testing

Allison Sindle, MD[a], Sharon E. Jacob, MD[b,c],*, Kari Martin, MD[a]

KEYWORDS

- Allergic contact dermatitis • Patch testing • Pediatric • Common allergens • Sensitization

KEY POINTS

- Pediatric allergic contact dermatitis (Ped-ACD) is an increasingly recognized highly prevalent skin disease, thought to be related to exposure to sensitizers at a young age or on an impaired skin barrier.
- Diagnosis of Ped-ACD can be challenging in the setting of other common pediatric skin diseases such as atopic dermatitis and irritant contact dermatitis.
- Knowledge of top pediatric allergens such as nickel, fragrance mix, cobalt, balsam of Peru, neomycin methylisothiazolinone, and formaldehyde releasing preservatives can aid in accurate diagnostic evaluation of pediatric patients with ACD.
- Specificity in allergen selection can lead to fewer false-positive (irritant reaction) results and increased probability of determining a true positive patch test reaction and a clinically relevant allergen.

INTRODUCTION

Pediatric allergic contact dermatitis [Ped-ACD] is an increasingly recognized highly prevalent skin disease that has a significant impact on the quality of life of patients and their families. Many patients presenting for patch testing have had chronic dermatitis for months to years, managed as other common pediatric skin diseases such as atopic dermatitis (AD) and irritant contact dermatitis (CD). Accurate and appropriate patch testing is critical in the diagnosis of Ped-ACD and requires knowledge of the most common allergens in the pediatric population, consideration of concurrent diseases that can complicate the clinical picture, and modification of techniques to lessen exposure to irritants and sensitizers while obtaining true positive results. This article reviews the most common pediatric allergens and discusses considerations when performing pediatric patch testing.

PEDIATRIC ALLERGIC CONTACT DERMATITIS

Allergic contact dermatitis (ACD) is a type IV delayed hypersensitivity reaction requiring primary sensitization and secondary elicitation response. It is the fifth most common skin disease and is estimated to affect approximately 13 million people in the United States, with 4.4 million of those being pediatric patients.[1] In pediatric patients, increased exposure to sensitizers at a young age or to an impaired barrier (eg, AD) may be a contributing

[a] Department of Dermatology, University of Missouri, 1 Hospital Drive, Room MA111, Columbia, MO 65212, USA; [b] Department of Medicine and Pediatrics, University of California, Riverside, 900 University Avenue, Riverside, CA 92521, USA; [c] Department of Dermatology, Loma Linda University, VA Loma Linda, Loma Linda, CA, USA
* Corresponding author. Department of Medicine and Pediatrics, University of California, Riverside, 900 University Avenue, Riverside, CA 92521.
E-mail address: sjacob@contactderm.net

Dermatol Clin 38 (2020) 321–327
https://doi.org/10.1016/j.det.2020.02.003

factor in the increasing diagnosis rate of pediatric ACD.[2] Historically, Ped-ACD was thought to be uncommon because of limited allergen exposure and an immature immune system. Repeated studies, however, have demonstrated contact sensitivity (reactivity on patch testing) in patients as young as 6 months of age.[3,4] Furthermore, repeated clinical trends demonstrate pediatric patients are sensitized to clinically relevant allergens because of exposures to medicaments, personal hygiene products, body piercings, sports-related gear, and certain hobbies.[2]

Data from the Pediatric Contact Dermatitis Registry (PCDR) showed an allergen sensitization rate of 13% to 25% in currently asymptomatic children,[5] supporting the prior evidence of significant sensitization in children. Furthermore, this study found that 65% of the tested pediatric patients had a positive patch result, with 48% of those being clinically relevant positive patch tests.[5] Along this same line, the North American Contact Dermatitis Group (NACDG) data from 2014 reported that 62.3% of patch-tested children had positive patch test results, and 56.7% of symptomatic children had a clinically relevant positive patch test result.[5,6] It is important to note that both studies demonstrated a significant sensitization rate in patients with AD. The NACDG reported that 48.3% of the pediatric patients with clinically relevant patch tests also carried the diagnosis of AD.[5] Notably, in concordance, Goldenberg and colleagues[3] reported that children with positive patch tests were 3 times as likely to have coexisting AD. This provides supporting evidence that the impaired epidermal barrier allows increased allergen penetration and subsequent sensitization and that patients with AD are at an increased risk for ACD.[3]

COMMON PEDIATRIC ALLERGENS
Top Allergens and Comparisons Between Pediatric and Adult Populations

In pediatric patch testing, it is important to consider exposures that are common in the pediatric population that may differ from common allergens seen in the adult population. The most common allergen in both populations is nickel.[3] To determine the most common allergens in children, a retrospective analysis of pediatric patch test results was performed from 2015 to 2016 for the PCDR.[5] The top 10 most common allergens from the analysis are nickel sulfate, fragrance mix I, cobalt, balsam of Peru, neomycin, propylene glycol, cocamidopropyl betaine, bacitracin, formaldehyde, and gold. Additional data sets have shown high prevalence and clinical relevance to methylisothiazolinone, paraphenylenediamine, cobalt chloride, and quaternium-15.[3,6] The most frequently encountered allergens in both pediatric and adult populations are compared in **Table 1**.[7,8]

Worldwide, the most common positive and clinically relevant allergens were nickel sulfate and cobalt chloride.[6] Common exposures related to these top allergens are piercings, orthodontic braces, coin rolling, school chairs, and ballet dance bars.[9] In Europe, prevalence of nickel allergy is 8% to 10% of the pediatric population, higher in patients with known dermatitis (5%–30%).[10] Countries such as Denmark, Sweden, Germany, and England have adopted regulations for nickel exposure because of the high prevalence. The European Union Nickel Directive regulates the amount of nickel content allowed to be released from products that may come into direct and prolonged contact with the skin.[10] In 2014, the European Chemicals Agency further specified that prolonged

Table 1
Most prevalent allergens with clinical relevance in pediatric and adult populations

	Pediatric	Adult
1	Nickel sulfate and cobalt chloride	Nickel sulfate
2	Fragrance mix I	Methylisothiazolinone
3	Balsam of Peru	Fragrance mix I
4	Neomycin sulfate	Formaldehyde 2%
5	Bacitracin	Methylchloroisothiazolinone/methylisothiazolinone
6	Wool (wax) alcohols	Balsam of Peru
7	Formaldehyde 1%	Neomycin
8	Methylisothiazolinone	Bacitracin
9	Bronopol	Formaldehyde 1%
10	Propylene glycol	Paraphenylenediamine

Comparison of the top 10 pediatric allergens from the P.E.A.S. (Pre-emptive Avoidance Strategy) analysis of PCDR & NACDG data,[7] and the top 10 adult allergens (2015–2016) from the NACDG data.[8]

contact was defined as "more than 10 minutes on three or more occasions within 2 weeks, or 30 minutes on one or more occasions within two weeks.[11]" It was later proven that short and repeated contact with the skin, especially in irritated sites/sites with prior dermatitis, can elicit ACD.[11]

After initiation of the regulations in Denmark, there was noted to be a significant decrease in the prevalence in nickel allergy, especially in young females.[12] Despite this decrease, however, approximately 10% of young women were found to be nickel allergic. Further studies showed a positive association between filaggrin null mutation status and nickel allergy; however, environmental nickel exposure was felt to be the leading cause of persistent allergy.[12] It is important to recognize the impact of concomitant AD in the sensitization of pediatric populations, as chronic exposure to weak allergens may result in sensitization. Conversely, because strong sensitizers such as MI are considered dependent upon a Th1-mediated response, patients with AD are considered to be less prone to sensitization because of an increased Th2/Th1 ratio.[4]

Common Allergens and Where to Find Them

Metals
Worldwide data demonstrate that nickel and cobalt are the top 2 pediatric allergens encountered in clinical practice. Several examples of common exposures have been discussed previously including piercing-associated jewelry allergy, orthodontics, school chairs, and equipment associated with hobbies (eg, ballet bars and sports equipment). Other common exposures include toys with metal components, instruments, electronics such as cell phones or video games, and metal fasteners in clothing.[13]

Topical antibiotics
Both neomycin and bacitracin are commonly used over the counter in the United States, often together, for minor injuries. Societal support for self-administration of topical antibiotics in the United States has led to children being sensitized at a young age, leading to these allergens landing in the top 10. Interestingly, neomycin has remained in the top pediatric allergens for over 3 decades.[13]

Fragrances
Fragrances are used to evoke or remove the sense of smell. Commonly used fragrances are fragrance mixes (I and II) and balsam of Peru, both of which are present in the top 10 pediatric and adult allergens. Balsam of Peru is an organic tree sap and as such contains a large number of volatile substances; several cross-react with other substituents found in foods (eg, cinnamic alcohol and tomatoes). Certain

spices such as cinnamon, vanilla, cloves, and anise, in addition to foods such as citrus fruits, soft drinks, and ketchup can lead to a systemic CD in persons sensitized to balsam of Peru.[13] Another example of a food-related fragrance is cinnamic aldehyde, which is present in cinnamon-flavored products/foods and can lead to a perioral or systemic dermatitis.[13] Common cross-reactive allergens with fragrances include propolis (derived from bee hives and present in lip balms and moisturizers) and colophony (derived from pine tree sap and present in adhesives, paper products, and shoes), which may be compounded together in products.[13]

Preservatives
Formaldehyde and its releasers are commonly used preservatives with antimicrobial properties. They are present in a significant number of cosmetic and personal care products. In the pediatric population, commonly used products with formaldehyde releasers include wet wipes, shampoos, and body washes.[13] Quaternium-15, a formaldehyde releaser, is a top 10 pediatric allergen.

Common nonformaldehyde preservatives include MCI and MI, which are becoming increasingly more common in the pediatric population with their presence in wet wipes, shampoos/washes, sunscreen, and homemade slime.[13] Other nonformaldehyde preservatives include parabens (that have low allergenic potential) and iodopropynyl butylcarbamate.

Surfactants
Surfactants (detergents) are widely encountered components of personal care products such as soaps and shampoos. Cocamidopropyl betaine [CAPB] is encountered frequently in the pediatric population, with its presence in no tear washes and shampoos.[9,13] It is so common an allergen found in patients with AD that some authors have stated that "Patients with AD should avoid the use of skincare products containing the surfactant CAPB."[14]

CONSIDERATIONS WHEN PERFORMING PEDIATRIC PATCH TESTING

When performing patch testing in the pediatric population, it is necessary to have a basic knowledge of the most commonly encountered allergens. There are several other considerations (eg, concurrent skin diseases) that can complicate the clinical picture and potential technique modifications to lessen exposure to irritants and sensitizers while obtaining true positive results.

Clinical Presentation

Pediatric ACD may present as a localized dermatitis, nonspecific pruritus, and scattered, generalized dermatitis. Shorter-duration dermatitis or new-onset dermatitis has a higher association with ACD in children.[5] Data from the PCDR showed that dermatitis of the ears was 10 times more likely to be associated with ACD to nickel than all other anatomic sites. Dermatitis of the face has also been frequently associated with ACD in relation to goggles/other equipment, fragranced products, and metals (such as cellular phones).[15] In pediatric patients with systemic CD, it is important to consider propylene glycol (present in oral suspension medications and processed foods) and balsam of Peru (a fragrance marker that cross-reacts with a significant number of base chemicals in natural foods); common triggers in children are chocolate or ketchup. Consideration should also be given to allergen exposure through caregiver contact (eg, mother's perfume or recently dyed hair).[15] It is beneficial for caregivers to bring objects and topical products used daily for evaluation and possible testing when considering patch placement.

In addition to predilection for specific sites, there appear to be differences in both gender and ethnic groups. ACD is more common in females, which is thought to be related to increased rates of sensitization through jewelry (nickel) and cosmetic products (fragrance).[5,16] Hispanic and Asian children are 2 times more likely than other ethnic groups to be diagnosed with ACD, which is attributed to different cultural practices and tendencies,[5] but also may be because of potential delays in evaluative care.

Lastly, age should be taken into consideration when evaluating a pediatric patient for ACD. Children under 5 years of age commonly become sensitized to personal hygiene products and are more likely to react to compositae mix than older children,[5] while children from age 6 to 18 years are most likely to be sensitized to allergens contained in their environment such as disperse blue and gold.[5] Furthermore, in evaluating CD in children it is important to consider allergens associated with sports equipment, musical instruments, school affects, and electronic devices when gathering pertinent history in the clinical encounter. Consideration of differences in exposures can guide allergen selection and determination of clinical relevance in the setting of a positive patch test. In a recent review, a set of guidelines was given to aid clinicians in determining the appropriate time to perform patch testing (**Box 1**).[1]

Concurrent Skin Disease

Evaluation in the setting of multifactorial pediatric dermatitis may be challenging, as many common skin diseases appear similar in presentation and may have concurrent expression. Examples

---

Box 1
Clinical scenarios in which clinicians should consider patch testing

Consider patch testing if:

- A patient's dermatitis increases in severity, changes distribution, does not improve with standard therapy, or quickly recurs after discontinuation of therapy
- A patient has a unique distribution of dermatitis
- A patient in the workforce has recalcitrant hand dermatitis (teens)
- A patient has adolescent-onset AD without prior history of childhood AD
- A patient has severe, widespread dermatitis that could require immunosuppressive medications, or has been repeatedly treated with systemic steroids

From Borok J, Matiz C, Goldenberg A, et al. Contact dermatitis in atopic dermatitis children-past, present, and future. Clin Rev Allergy Immunol 2019;56(1):86-98; with permission.

---

include AD, irritant CD, seborrheic dermatitis, and nummular dermatitis.

In a recent review of PCDR data, it was determined that 49% of patients with positive patch testing had a history of AD and 30% had a concurrent known diagnosis.[5,17] These patients typically presented for patch testing at a younger age and were more likely to present with a generalized dermatitis.[1] Concurrent AD confounds the clinical picture and has the potential to alter rates and the prevalence of contact sensitizers, increasing the risk of developing ACD. Patients with AD have decreased barrier function, leading to altered absorption of chemicals across the barrier and increased sensitization to certain allergens. Common allergens in this population include cocamidopropyl betaine, wool alcohol, lanolin, tixocortol pivalate, and parthenolide (a component of compositae). Many of these products are used daily in AD patients in topical medications and skin care products.[1,17]

When evaluating patients with concurrent skin disease such as AD, it is important to obtain a thorough history and physical examination. Suspicion for ACD is increased when there is development of a new-onset dermatitis in a patient with chronic dermatitis, or increased body surface area.[5] In addition, recalcitrant dermatitis despite adherence to treatment recommendations should prompt further investigation for ACD.[3] Untreated ACD can lead to chronic pruritus, sleep disturbances for the child and the family, secondary infections, economic burden, social stigma, and absence from work or school.[2,3] These factors have a profound impact on the quality of lives of both patients and their families.

Diagnostic Modifications

After considering the possibility of differences in clinical presentation and concurrent skin diseases, it is important to ensure accurate, quality patch testing. When considering patch testing in a pediatric patient, necessary factors are determination of body surface area available for testing, specification in allergen selection, potential reduction in allergy concentration, or exposure time modifications to the patch testing procedure.

In children, the body surface area available for patch placement is significantly smaller in size than that of adults. Because of this, there are limitations in the overall number of patches that can be placed. There is no standardized guideline on the correct number of allergens/patches to be placed when comprehensively evaluating a pediatric patient, as all reasonably suspected allergens deserve evaluation. That said, it is critical that the allergens be appropriately placed without risk for self-removal. In a 2- to 4-year-old patient, the average number of allergens that can be placed per average surface area on the

back is 40 to 45,[4] while the back of a 6- to 8-year-old patient may easily accommodate 60 to 80 allergens. Because of these space limitations, it is important to use the history and physical examination in the guidance and selection of the most suspected allergens for patch testing, as these would likely cover the greatest clinical relevance (and potential for remission with guided avoidance) in the patient. Specificity in allergen selection is also important for reducing false positives, or irritant reactions.[5]

Determining which allergens to test can be challenging for clinicians. In 2017, the thin-layer rapid-use epicutaneous patch (T.R.U.E. TEST, SmartPractice, Phoenix, Arizona) test was approved by the US Food and Drug Administration (FDA) for patch testing in children aged 6 to 18 years. This test contains 35 commonly encountered allergen components (and 1 negative control) and may serve as a basic screening tool; however, highly relevant allergens are not included in the kit (eg, cocamidopropyl betaine), while others are have a high false-negative rate (eg, methylisothiazolinone).[9] In 1 study, 39% of pediatric patients had relevant positive patch tests to allergens that were not included in the T.R.U.E. TEST.[18] In an effort to expand on this test and provide a

Table 2
Pediatric baseline series

Nickel sulfate	Carba mix
Quaternium-15	Imidazolidinyl urea
Neomycin	Lanolin
Balsam of Peru	Compositae mix
Fragrance mix I	Cinnamic aldehyde
MCI/MI	Paraben mix
Bacitracin	Thiuram mix
Propylene glycol	Bronopol
MI	Sesquiterpene lactones
Fragrance mix II	Colophony
Cocamidopropyl betaine	p-tert-Butylphenol-formaldehyde resin
Cobalt chloride	Clobetasol-17-propionate
Formaldehyde	Decyl glucoside
Propolis	Iodopropynyl butylcarbamate
Tixocortol-21-pivalate	Benzophenone-3
Hydrocortisone-17-butyrate	Amidoamine
Diazolidinyl urea	Tea tree oil
DMDM hydantoin	Carmine
Budesonide	Dimethylaminopropylamine

Abbreviations: MCI, methylchloroisothiazolinone; MI, methylisothiazolinone.
Components of proposed pediatric baseline series that captures the most common allergens encountered in pediatric patch testing.
Data from Yu J, Atwater A, Brod B, et al. Pediatric baseline patch test series: pediatric contact dermatitis workgroup. Dermatitis 2018;29(4):206–12.

pediatric baseline series, Yu and colleagues[13] conducted surveys and workgroups with patch testing professionals to determine the most commonly encountered pediatric allergens that would be of greatest benefit to include in a pediatric baseline patch testing series. The workgroup suggested 38 allergens be considered for inclusion in a basic pediatric screening series (**Table 2**).

Because of an increased body surface area to volume ratio in young children, there is the potential for increased relative absorption of topical preparations. It is important, especially in children younger than 8 years (age at which most children reach 75% of their adult body surface area to volume ratio[5]), to either consider modifying concentrations of allergens or time interval for exposure during patch testing.[3] Specific allergens in which modifications were recommended by Fisher include nickel, formaldehyde, and rubber additives.[19] Evidence from the last decade from the German Contact Dermatitis Research Group[20] and several United States-based groups have adopted the measure of decreased exposure to 24 hours (with reads at 48 and 72–120 hours) for children younger than 8 years of age, and the resulting true positive patch test results have been comparable.[4,20] On the other hand, for children older than 12 years of age, a typical adult patch testing procedure can be employed (removal at 48 hours, with reads at 96 and 120 hours).

A psychosocial tool that has been used to help young children cope with the patch test experience (sitting through an extensive consultation and diagnostic patch test evaluation), is video distraction assist. Using techniques to distract pediatric patients through play or developing a rewards system improves the patch placement and evaluation experience by reducing stress.[4,15] Counseling parents on techniques to reinforce the importance of keeping patches in place is crucial. Because of the significant increase in the detection rates of clinically relevant allergens, consideration of using repeat open application testing (R.O.A.T.) with the patient's personal hygiene products should be considered in conjunction with conventional patch testing.[4]

SUMMARY

With the increasing prevalence of Ped-ACD, it is becoming even more crucial to consider this diagnosis in pediatric patients with chronic, generalized, or recalcitrant dermatitis. Rapid evaluation will lead to decreased time to resolution and increased quality of life for patients and their families. Remaining up to date on the most common pediatric allergens in conjunction with clinical decision-making based on a thorough history and physical examination will

lead to selective patch testing. Selective patch testing allows increased probability of determining the causative allergen and decreased risk of false-positive results. As these techniques are employed, pediatric ACD will be diagnosed earlier and more accurately.

DISCLOSURE

A. Sindle and K. Martin have nothing to disclose. S.E. Jacob is the CEO of Dermatitis Academy, a webucation company dedicated to CD education.

REFERENCES

1. Borok J, Matiz C, Goldenberg A, et al. Contact dermatitis in atopic dermatitis children - past, present, and future. Clin Rev Allergy Immunol 2019;56:86–98.
2. Ascha M, Irfan M, Bena J, et al. Pediatric patch testing: a 10-year retrospective study. Ann Allergy Asthma Immunol 2016;117:661–7.
3. Goldenberg A, Silverberg N, Silverberg J, et al. Pediatric allergic contact dermatitis: lessons for better care. J Allergy Clin Immunol Pract 2015;3:661–7.
4. Sung C, McGowan M, Jacob S. Allergic contact dermatitis evaluation: strategies for the preschooler. Curr Allergy Asthma Rep 2018;10:49.
5. Goldenberg A, Mousdicas N, Silverberg N, et al. Pediatric contact dermatitis registry inaugural case data. Dermatitis 2016;27(5):293–302.
6. Zug K, Pham A, Belsito D, et al. Patch testing in children from 2005 to 2012: results from the North American Contact Dermatitis Group. Dermatitis 2014;25(6):345–55.
7. Brankov N, Jacob S. Pre-emptive avoidance strategy 2016: update on pediatric contact dermatitis allergens. Expert Rev Clin Immunol 2016;13(2):93–5.
8. DeKoven J, Warshaw E, Zug K, et al. North American contact dermatitis group patch test results: 2015-2016. Dermatitis 2018;29(6):297–309.
9. Jacob S, Brod B, Crawford G. Clinically relevant patch test reactions in children - a United States based study. clinical and laboratory investigations. Pediatr Dermatol 2008;25(6):520–7.
10. Ahlstrom M, Thyssen J, Wennervaldt M, et al. Nickel allergy and allergic contact dermatitis: a clinical review of immunology, epidemiology, exposure, and treatment. Contact Dermatitis 2019;81(4):227–41.
11. Ahlstrom M, Thyssen J, Menne T, et al. Short contact with nickel causes allergic contact dermatitis: an experimental study. Br J Dermatol 2018;179:1127–34.
12. Thyssen J. Nickel and cobalt allergy before and after nickel regulation – evaluation of a public health intervention. Contact Dermatitis 2011;65(1):1–68.
13. Yu J, Atwater A, Brod B, et al. Pediatric baseline patch test series: pediatric contact dermatitis workgroup. Dermatitis 2018;29(4):206–12.
14. Shaughnessy C, Malajian D, Belsito D. Cutaneous delayed-type hypersensitivity in patients with atopic

dermatitis: reactivity to surfactants. J Am Acad Dermatol 2014;70(4):704–8.

15. Brod B, Treat J, Rothe M, et al. Allergic contact dermatitis: kids are not just little people. Clin Dermatol 2015;33:605–12.

16. Warshaw E, Aschenbeck K, DeKoven J, et al. Epidemiology of pediatric nickel sensitivity: Retrospective review of North American Contact Dermatitis Group (NACDG) data 1994-2014. J Am Acad Dermatol 2018;79(4):664–71.

17. Jacob S, McGowan M, Silverberg N, et al. Pediatric contact dermatitis registry data on contact allergy in children with atopic dermatitis. JAMA Dermatol 2017;153(8):765–70.

18. Zug K, McGinley-Smith D, Washaw E, et al. Contact allergy in children referred for patch testing. Arch Dermatol 2008;144(10):1329–36.

19. Admani S, Jacob S. Allergic contact dermatitis in children: review of the past decade. Curr Allergy Asthma Rep 2014;14:421.

20. Worm M, Aberer W, Agathos M, et al. Patch testing in children - recommendations of the German Contact Dermatitis Research Group. J Dtsch Dermatol Ges 2007;5:107–9.

Occupational Contact Dermatitis
Evaluation and Management Considerations

Lauren Claire Hollins, MD, Alexandra Flamm, MD*

KEYWORDS

- Contact dermatitis • Allergic contact dermatitis • Irritant contact dermatitis
- Occupational contact dermatitis • Management • Evaluation • Patch testing
- Workers compensation

KEY POINTS

- Occupational contact dermatitis is commonly encountered among workers, particularly those in wet work.
- Eighty percent of occupational contact dermatitis is due to irritant contact dermatitis and the remaining 20% is categorized as allergic contact dermatitis.
- An accurate diagnosis by the dermatologist relies on meticulous physical examination and inquisitive history taking.
- Comprehensive patch testing is the gold standard for diagnosing allergic contact dermatitis.
- Although occupational contact dermatitis management represents a challenge to the dermatologist, it can be achieved with attention to detail and appropriate patient follow-up.

INTRODUCTION

Contact dermatitis in the workplace is responsible for most skin disease in the industrialized world, accounting for up to 90% of occupational skin disorders.[1] It is also likely underreported, especially in mild cases, and a recent survey of more than 27,000 adults determined that the overall prevalence of dermatitis was 9.8%, representing more than 15 million affected US workers.[2] Occupational contact dermatitis (OCD) can be divided broadly into irritant contact dermatitis (ICD) and allergic contact dermatitis (ACD). ICD makes up the vast majority, approximately 80% of OCD, whereas ACD encompasses the remaining percentage. However in many cases, ACD and ICD are present concomitantly, especially on exposed parts of the body, such as the hands.[1] To make an accurate diagnosis, the dermatologist must work deliberately and slowly to acquire a detailed history, perform a thorough physical examination, and carefully interpret data obtained about the workplace. At times, a work site visit is helpful to further gather crucial data and corroborate the diagnosis. This article provides an overview of how to evaluate a patient, perform a workplace visit, and properly manage this potentially frustrating diagnosis, both for the worker and the dermatologist.

EVALUATION CONSIDERATIONS

OCD is responsible for almost all cutaneous reactions that happen in the workplace, and has the potential to significantly impact the quality of life in those affected.[3] It encompasses a wide range of clinical manifestations from various potential exposures, typically depending on the patient's category of work. The most important parts of determining the cause of a worker's rash are in

Department of Dermatology, Penn State Health, Milton S. Hershey Medical Center, 500 University Drive, Hershey, PA 17033, USA
* Corresponding author.
E-mail address: aflamm@pennstatehealth.psu.edu

Dermatol Clin 38 (2020) 329–338
https://doi.org/10.1016/j.det.2020.02.001
0733-8635/20/© 2020 Elsevier Inc. All rights reserved.

the evaluation of the patient, the collecting of data, which may or may not include a patch test, and potentially conducting a site visit.

The Office Visit

Many patients present to a health care provider as a first step in the evaluation of their rash. The referral to a dermatology clinic may come from the patient themselves, their employer, a primary care physician, an occupational medicine physician, or an insurer. The time allotted for this initial visit is crucial to gathering information, and an extended appointment will likely be required to gather the proper history, discuss possible exposures and perform the physical examination.

The History

A detailed elicitation of the patient history begins the diagnostic quest, including the timing, location of the rash, and change in the rash in relation to work (ie, improvement away from work with worsening upon return heightens suspicion that the dermatitis is work related). A detailed discussion of the description of the work is also important. The dermatologist will want to know what potential contactants are used, what the patient believes they are exposed to, and whether or not they have access to information about the composition of these materials. Encourage patients to bring these data with them to the appointment if available. One Canadian survey of dermatologists revealed that only 5% of dermatologists inquired about exposures and only 3% asked patients to bring Material Safety Data Sheets (MSDSs; now referred to as Safety Data Sheets [SDSs]) from the workplace to the clinic visit.[4] Also inquire about physical symptoms. If the patient describes burning, erythema, or stinging, these findings may be suggestive of irritant dermatitis, potentially negating the need for a patch test. However, if the patient notes intense, intractable pruritus, this may be indicative of ACD. Another important question to ask is whether or not the patient is currently taking oral corticosteroids, or any other immunosuppressive medications, which may dampen the results of patch testing, if a patch test is required.[5] Patients can take oral antihistamines as needed for symptoms because they should not alter patch test results.[6]

You will also want to know about the patient's past medical history. Do they have a history of atopy, hay fever, or self-described sensitive skin? These questions can point to a history of atopic dermatitis (AD). AD results in an impairment of the skin barrier, for involved as well as uninvolved skin, and it can result in increased absorption of allergens when exposed to chemicals.[7] It should be noted that the questions mentioned elsewhere in this article will not rule in or out whether the present rash is ACD or an atopic flare. That must be done by the physical examination and, if needed, a patch test.

Perhaps the most important part of history taking is the occupational history. Sometimes, the rash has resolved when the patient presents in clinic (eg, difficulty scheduling or time spent away from work). Therefore, the physician must work as a detective to elicit proper information. The exact timeline of a typical day at work from arrival to departure should be elicited, as well as dates the rash began. This information is helpful not only to determine the causative allergen, but it is important legally for the employer. If the patient has the rash at all times, whether on extended vacations or working, then the symptoms are less likely to be due to work exposures. Details about the work site, the daily tasks the job entails, products used in restrooms if known, personal protective equipment and if other coworkers are affected should be elicited. Distribution of the rash is also paramount. Simplified, repeated questions may be needed, because it is likely that many patients will not think to discuss the daily and routine actions performed at work, such as exposure to contaminated water from leaking pipes or the regular protective gear used in the work area. Finally, inquire about treatments used, including prescriptions, over-the-counter medications, and home remedies.

The steps to acquiring this history may take time, so it is appropriate to schedule 1 appointment solely for obtaining a detailed history. It is also appropriate to schedule a longer appointment, to obtain the history, perform the physical examination, and potentially place patches. It is likely that the patient may have to drive far distances for this appointment, so minimizing travel time with 1, longer visit is ideal.

Even with a detailed history, the diagnosis for OCD is often difficult because no one clinical or dermatopathologic finding is characteristic. Criteria have been proposed to help guide the practitioner to the correct diagnosis if OCD is suspected, named the Mathias criteria (**Table 1**).[8] The 7 criteria proposed by Mathias assess the probability for workplace causality. Responding yes to at least 4 items suggests that there is greater than 50% probability of occupational causation, implying a reasonable degree of medical certainty that the dermatitis is workplace induced. The criteria has been validated, which is helpful as it can be used to help build a case for workers' compensation, which is discussed elsewhere in this article.[9]

Table 1
Summary of the Mathias criteria for assessing occupational causation and/or aggravation of contact dermatitis

Criterion 1	Is the clinical appearance consistent with contact dermatitis?
Criterion 2	Are there workplace exposures to potential cutaneous irritants or allergens?
Criterion 3	Is the anatomic distribution of dermatitis consistent with cutaneous exposure in relation to the job task?
Criterion 4	Is the temporal relationship between exposure and onset consistent with contact dermatitis?
Criterion 5	Are nonoccupational exposures excluded as probable causes?
Criterion 6	Does dermatitis improve away from work exposure to the suspected irritant or allergen?
Criterion 7	Do patch or provocation tests identify a probable causal agent?

Data from Clark SC, Zirwas MJ. Management of Occupational Dermatitis. *Dermatol Clin.* 2009;27(3):365-383. https://doi.org/10.1016/j.det.2009.05.002.

The Physical Examination

Once the history is elicited, the physical examination and, if needed, patch placement, can be performed. First, the provider should ensure that the patient is in a gown with all affected skin easily accessible. During a full skin examination, look for corroborating evidence to the patient's history, and also make note of the distribution of the dermatitis. In classical airborne contact dermatitis, look for areas of involvement that can help to differentiate between photo-related dermatitis such as underneath the chin, the eyelids, and any other exposed skin of concern.[10] It is also important to assess the morphology of the lesions. Lichenified plaques can denote chronicity, whereas weeping, bullous plaques can lead one to think of a more acute process (**Table 2**).

After assessing the exposed skin for dermatitis, confirm that the patient's skin is clear enough for patch placement. This step is important to ensure accurate interpretation of the results. Do not hesitate to perform a potassium hydroxide preparation to evaluate for dermatophytosis or skin biopsy as needed to avoid unnecessary treatments.

Patch testing, the cornerstone of diagnosing ACD, is a cost-effective test with a sensitivity and specificity of 70% to 80%.[11] Be mindful that it is only helpful if there is a strong suspicion for ACD and if the allergens that are tested will be relevant to potential occupational exposures.[12] If a patch test is warranted owing to suspicion of ACD, discuss with the patient about what to expect with the results and set expectations. After patches have been placed, the appropriate interval for reading must be adhered to. Patches should be left in place for at least 48 to 72 hours from the date of initial application, ensuring proper contact time for the allergens to react. It is important to provide patients with written instructions for

Table 2
Distinguishing features of ICD and ACD

Feature	ICD	ACD
Pathogenesis	Direct cytotoxicity, skin barrier disruption. Does not require sensitization to allergen.	Activation of allergen-specific T cells; delayed hypersensitivity. Requires sensitization to allergen.
Concentration of contactant	High.	Low.
Affected	Anyone and everyone.	A minority of patients.
Clinical features	Subacute to chronic eczema with fissuring, scaling, erythema.	Acute to subacute eczema, occasionally with weeping, bullae, or vesicles.
Patient complaint	Pain or burning.	Pruritus.
Onset	Immediately.	Slowly; after initial sensitization, 12–48 h to elicitation of dermatitis.
Diagnosis	History and physical examination.	History and physical examination, patch testing.

when they go home, stressing that they should refrain from showering, because doing so can make the patch test results difficult to interpret. At 48 hours, the patches can be removed and interpreted for a first reading. The second reading can take place 24 hours after the first reading, to allow slower allergens to develop. Some allergens do require more time to develop beyond the typical time frame that a clinician would read results. A recent study noted additional readings after day 7 were useful for identifying reactions to many metals, including gold and cobalt; some preservatives such as propolis; and the topical antibiotic neomycin.[13] Therefore, patients should be adequately counseled on delayed reactions and alert the dermatologist if they become symptomatic. Alternatively, it may be helpful to schedule a follow-up visit in the appropriate time interval for a manual check.

Sometimes the patient may bring their own allergen sample for testing, but be cautious because the substance may be caustic, and it may need to be diluted to avoid potentially severe reactions like ulceration and infection if applied directly to the skin. Published guidelines are available to help mix potential allergens to appropriate levels and should be consulted in these situations.[14]

Performing a Site Visit

At times, an actual site visit may be required. This can be the case when multiple persons are affected, if the patient history is unclear, or if doing a site visit is requested by the employer. A site visit is helpful because the dermatologist can perform a thorough walkthrough, including breakrooms, bathrooms, and other indirect locations. A site visit is also helpful because it allows the physician to become familiar with work conditions and to understand the work environment of a site.

Perhaps the best way to arrange a visit is to call the site manager or occupational medicine specialist associated with the company. In this way, you can establish relationships and navigate through proper protocols for a visit. Sometimes, special shoes or garments are required, and proper sizing will need to be obtained before beginning the visit. Any discussion of compensation should be discussed with appropriate persons before scheduling the visit, although it should be noted that the dermatologist can perform these visits free of charge; one should be mindful of potential lost revenue if running a practice.

Once a date for the visit has been established, plan for at least a half day. This amount of time will be enough to do a proper visit and meet with necessary involved persons. At the start of a visit, it is common to meet with a human resources representative, who may provide a presentation or overview of events surrounding the dermatitis, which can be quite helpful to corroborate patient narratives.

Meeting with officials is also helpful to obtain the names of the chemicals and potential allergens in question, if not previously provided by the worker. They will likely provide SDSs, which are documents providing information regarding hazardous materials or mixtures present on site. More details about SDSs are discussed elsewhere in this article. At this time, one can meet with other workers who may have also had dermatitis but could not come to clinic. Keep in mind that no question is too simple; ask basic questions that provide information on how machines work, how they are maintained, start and end times for shifts, and whether or not workers on different shifts have similar rashes, for example.

After initial meetings and oftentimes after donning appropriate protective gear, a walkthrough of the facility will be performed. This step is as crucial to the site visit as a physical examination is to a clinic visit. This is the time for the physician to look closely at the work environment, make assessments, ask real-time questions, and take notes. Many observations can be made: What do the employees wear to protect their skin? How many workers are in an area? If time allows, it is ideal to act as a "fly on the wall" for at least a portion of the visit to get as close to unbiased data as possible. The cleanliness of the area and potential exposures, such as materials from leaks, spills, and contaminated surfaces, should be documented. Make time to evaluate common areas like bathrooms and breakrooms. Take note of the ingredients in hand cleansers, the use of disinfecting wipes used by staff, and other potential discoveries.

After the walkthrough is completed, have a wrap-up session with the involved parties. This is a time to meet with everyone again and debrief. A summary should be provided at the end of the visit, and at that time it can be decided if a formal write-up is needed. A timeline should be provided to the site to set expectations. Finally, obtain contact information for all relevant parties in case new evidence becomes available.

MANAGEMENT CONSIDERATIONS: PREVENTION AND THERAPY
Prevention

Prevention is the foundation of managing occupational dermatitis. After the cause of the dermatitis is determined, education for affected workers is paramount. Education involves patient recognition of hazardous materials and the various names under which allergens can be listed as ingredients. Because some allergens that are found in work environments may also be found in home products, it is important to relay this information clearly to workers. Providing patients with a list of products that are devoid of allergens is helpful. The American Contact Dermatitis Society maintains the Contact Allergen Management Program for members, an online service that will list all products that do not contain the allergens in question. Free videos that describe some allergens are available at www.contactdermatitisinstitute.com; other databases listing products are also available for a fee.

Information must be provided for the patient to make changes in products used and for the worksite to make updates to its safety protocols and products used (eg, changing the cleanser in the restrooms). When discussing with the patient, information must also be presented in a way that is easily understood and concise, keeping in mind the various levels of education and health literacy in patients. The use of pictures on handouts is encouraged, as well as in-office demonstrations of label reading.[15] There are standardized patient education materials available from reputable resources such as the American Contact Dermatitis Society that can be accessed online. Caution must be used to avoid information overload, and it may be pertinent to bring the patient back for multiple appointments or provide access to a nurse or physician line for additional questions that may arise after leaving the clinic. Alternatively, it is reasonable to schedule a follow-up phone call if returns to clinic are not feasible.

Hazard Control

Safety data sheets
Ensuring that all hazardous materials are accounted for and controlled is imperative. SDSs, previously known as MSDSs, are documents and communications providing information concerning hazardous materials or mixtures present at a given worksite. Employers are required to have these data available, and all workers should be aware of the location and contents of the SDSs, or be able to request information. Before the 2012 switch, MSDSs frequently had little helpful information to the dermatologist. Ingredients were frequently not listed correctly, terms were often too general, and potential allergens were not listed at all if deemed unnecessary by the manufacturer. Because of these shortcomings,

the Occupational Safety and Health Administration implemented The Hazard Communication Standard to align with the Globally Harmonized System of Classification and Labeling of Chemicals. This updated system standardized chemical safety information, and improved on the MSDSs, thus improving workplace safety. Although the MSDS could include various levels of detail about chemicals, the SDS format is more in-depth and meets international standards. More information can be located from the United States Department of Labor website (osha.gov).

The employer and employee
The employer should be sure that the facility meets safety codes, and that all employees are aware of SDSs, accident protocols, and how to report them correctly. Ventilation of the work environment should be proper and regulated by correct governing bodies to avoid airborne OCD. Access to detailed accounts of maintenance reports should be available and up to date. Wash stations for splashes, drips, and spills should be visible, clean, and in working order.

Proper clothing, eye protection, and other necessary safety needs should be in place. It is important to ensure that these recommendations and protocols are done at the companywide level to help decrease the rate at which other workers may be affected. For the individual workers, following all protocols in place and consideration of appointing a safety liaison is helpful.

Gloves
It is known that hand dermatitis is seen in most cases of OCD and poses a large burden on workers owing to increased sick leave, job loss, and even early retirement.[16] Thus, appropriate glove use is critical for hand protection. The type of glove used depends heavily on the type of chemicals the gloves are meant to protect workers from, as well as their allergenic potential, and the skin exposure time, because many gloves that are billed as impermeable may eventually allow small amounts of chemical or irritant to leak through. Hand sweating can further contribute to existing dermatitis, so gloves should be changed frequently.[11] In addition, patients should be careful to avoid allergens becoming trapped in gloves accidently, exacerbating OCD. It should be remembered that actual glove materials have the potential to cause ACD or ICD. Permeation and degradation are types of chemical resistance properties that should be considered when selecting gloves, and some general glove characteristics are listed in **Table 3**.

Table 3
Summary of general characteristics of glove materials

Material	Chemical Protection		Biologic Protection	Puncture and Tear Resistance	Dexterity	Price	Allergy
	Good	Poor					
Latex	Water	Most chemicals	Excellent	Good	Excellent	Low	Type I, type IV
Nitrite	Water, most organic solvents, most hydrocarbons, oils, greases, selected acids and bases	Ketones, aromatics, chlorinated hydrocarbons, esters, some acids	Good	Good	Good	Low	Type IV
Vinyl	Acids, bases, oils, greases, peroxides, amines	Organic or petroleum based solvents, aldehydes	Poor	Poor	Poor	Low	Rare
Neoprene	Alcohols, phenols, peroxides, acids, hydrocarbons, bases	Halogenated and aromatic hydrocarbons	Good	Good	Good	Medium	Type IV
Multilayer laminates	All classes	Isolated small molecule solvents	N/A	Medium	Very poor	High	Rare

Material	Chemical Protection	Biologic Protection	Dexterity	Durability	Price	Allergy
Latex	Poor	Best	Best	Good	Low	Type I, type IV
Nitrite	Good	Good	Good	Good	Low	Type IV
Vinyl	Fair	Poor	Poor	Poor	Low	None
Neoprene	Good	Good	Good	Good	High	Uncommon

Data from Clark SC, Zirwas MJ. Management of Occupational Dermatitis. Dermatol Clin. 2009;27(3):365-383. https://doi.org/10.1016/j.det.2009.05.002.

Ointments and barrier creams

Ointments are the standard bearers of OCD prevention. They act as a protective layer, shielding the skin from potential irritants and allergens. Oil-based products provide the most protection; they repel paints, solvents, and other chemicals workers encounter. They have also been shown to be efficacious against water-based products like acids, alkalis, and metalworking fluids.[17] Historically, it has been difficult to prove the benefits of ointment skin protectants in OCD treatment.[18–20] Nevertheless, ointments are the authors' preferred vehicle for therapy. Barrier creams represent another option for prevention, albeit a controversial one, because some studies failed to find benefit.[21,22] A systematic review reported mixed evidence for the effectiveness of prework barrier creams,[23] but did conclude that barrier creams containing products such as dimethicone could help in preventing ICD. Winker and colleagues[22] found a benefit to barrier creams when used with mild cleansers and after work treatments. It is important to note that barrier creams themselves may cause allergic reactions, and should not be used on affected skin. Additionally, they must be applied frequently enough in adequate amounts to be effective.

Many patients prefer the relative cosmetic elegance of creams to ointment-based products. However, use of barrier creams should not be oversold as preventative treatment because they may confer a sense of security that is not warranted and could lead to a laxity in stringent preventive measures.[24]

Harsh soaps and degreasers

Patients should be educated on the potential irritation caused by harsh soaps and degreasers. If these products must be used, proper gloves must be worn, as discussed elsewhere in this article. If the skin is dry or even slightly irritated, a thick moisturizer should be used after hand washing.[25]

The workers should use the mildest cleansers available, as intermittently as possible, to avoid complications. Mild *synthetic* *de*tergents called "syndets" are commonly used replacements for true soaps. Closer to physiologic skin pH, syndets contain less than 10% soap and work to minimize cutaneous alkalinization.[26] Recognizable syndets include Dove (Unilever, London, UK) and Cetaphil (Galderma Laboratories, Fort Worth, TX).

The physician

The role of the physician lies most importantly in providing the correct diagnosis and, after the diagnosis is made, identification of the hazard so that it can be avoided. Worker education is also vital. The worker should be well-versed in their allergen and should know what to do if subsequently exposed. Providing safe lists as found through the Contact Allergen Management Program database can also be helpful because some allergens are found both in the workplace and at home. Patients must also understand the proper use and side effect profile of prescribed medications and general skin care tips. Printed handouts are helpful to relay information.

Therapies

Topical corticosteroids remain the cornerstone treatment for most cases of acute contact dermatitis, particularly ACD. Studies have documented the efficacy of topical steroids in ACD,[27,28] and their efficacy using even class II or III corticosteroids is undisputed.[29]

ICD has a somewhat less clear benefit from weaker preparations of topical steroid[29]; however, as associated inflammation is reduced, they are still recommended for acute relief. There have been reports of systemic absorption of corticosteroids from misused topical formulations[30]; therefore, steroids should be given in the correct strength and for the proper duration for the body site affected to avoid potential side effects.[31] Finally, some studies[32,33] have documented patient allergy to certain classes of topical steroids, so keep this in mind when treating patients who are not improving or worsening on appropriate topical therapy.

Systemic steroids can be used for brief periods, ideally less than 4 weeks, for extensive dermatitis, and sedative antihistamines can be used to help patients sleep through the night and potentially help with pruritus, and both treatments remain helpful adjuncts for OCD.

Topical calcineurin inhibitors (TCIs) have become important treatment options to help mitigate the side effects of chronic topical steroid use. After an initial topical and/or oral steroid burst to quell patient symptoms, TCIs can be used for maintenance as needed. A prospective study on hand dermatitis found comparable outcomes with use of tacrolimus 0.1% ointment compared with mometasone furoate for hand ACD.[34] Common side effects of topical TCIs include burning or a warm sensation, and both symptoms should resolve with consistent use. TCIs are a good option for OCD in sensitive locations such as the face and neck.

Crisaborole, a topical phosphodiesterase-4 inhibitor, is a newer therapy option; however, it is currently only approved by the US Food and Drug Administration for mild to moderate AD. However, because ACD represents a potential comorbidity and exacerbates AD,[35] the use of crisaborole can be considered in patients with a known diagnosis of AD and concomitant suspected or confirmed ACD.

Recommending a sensitive skin care routine to patients is essential. Patients should be directed to use gentle, nonsoap cleansers such as Cetaphil (Galderma Laboratories), CereVe (Coria Laboratories, Dallas, TX), or Vanicream (Pharmaceutical Specialties, Inc., Rochester, MD), which are void of many common allergens, but certainly direct patients to read the ingredient labels. Thick creams or ointments should be used after washing hands. Regular washing of contaminated clothing should be performed in unscented laundry detergent. It has been reported numerous times in the literature that alcohol-based, waterless hand sanitizers cause less irritation than traditional soap and water, and this should be discussed with workers and management teams as needed.

WORKERS' COMPENSATION

Workers' compensation laws were an instrumental development beginning in the early parts of the Industrial Revolution, as society moved from being mostly agricultural to predominantly industrial. First enacted in parts of Europe in the late 1800s, they became part of United States law in 1911. Before these laws, the employee or their representative sued the employer for damages, resulting in lengthy and expensive processes, and ultimately, put the worker at a major disadvantage. The principal idea behind workers' compensation laws ensure that employees have medical treatment and compensation without regard to fault, and that costs are assumed by the employer. Modern-day workers' compensation is an insurance that almost all employers must carry, and varies widely between states. According to the *Insurance Journal*, in a majority of states, a small business with even 1 employee must carry workers' compensation insurance, and if employers skip coverage, they are liable to hefty penalties. The percentage of a worker's compensated salary and/or the amount of work lost before benefits start also vary depending on the worker's state of residence. For these reasons, it is advisable for workers to consider retaining an attorney. In most cases, there are no upfront costs, and attorneys get fees from awarded workers' compensation benefits.

DISABILITY

Disability insurance is different from workers' compensation. Disability insurance functions similarly to health insurance. It can be purchased by individual workers for themselves, provided through Social Security Disability Insurance, or purchased from the worker's employer. Contrasting workers' compensation, disability is not reliant on workplace injury or illness, only on how severely the functional abilities of the worker are affected, no matter where the injury took place. The range is from totally disabled to partially or not disabled. In the case of Social Security Disability Insurance, a judge makes the decision. If the worker uses their insurance, the insurance company will determine disability, which depends on the details of the policy.

In summary, workers' compensation answers the question of whether or not a worker is injured as a direct result of their job, and that determination is based on occupational causality, which must be established. Disability describes whether or not an injury or illness is severe enough to limit the person's ability for gainful employment, without regard to how or where it occurred.

The Physician's Role

Often times, physicians must fill out a work abilities form, which reports on worker limitations, and these forms are used in part to determine workers' compensation or disability. This paperwork is important to fill out as accurately as possible, not only for good medical care and diagnosis, but also for the large impact it will have on the worker's economic and emotional well-being. Before filling out any forms, establishing a causal relationship between work and the skin condition is most important for the worker, albeit difficult to prove. The basis of the physician's findings are crucial here, because the place of employment may dispute the claim. Patch test results will oftentimes be critical and should be used if ACD is suspected. Positive patch test results that have workplace relevance are the most significant for establishing a causal relationship for workers' compensation. The timing of the rash in relation to work can also help to determine a relationship and aid in any difficult cases.

Physicians may have a potentially difficult role in workers' compensation claims. It should be noted that the more restrictions physicians place on the worker, the less likely the worker will be able to return to work. However, not placing enough restrictions can lead to the worker sustaining continuing injury.[24] Overall, the history and physical examination should lead the physician on any decision making with regards to the work abilities form.

Preparing a Letter and/or Report

A medical report will need to be drafted and should follow the same format as any letter to a referring physician. However, it is important to take into consideration that this letter needs to be understood and interpreted by workers, employers, and disability and workers' compensation personnel, and should be written in nonphysician terms. The letter should include the history and physical examination, patch test results, site visit findings, results of follow-up clinic visits, and physician recommendations. As described by Clark and Zirwas,[24] the report may also include the following if desired: (1) an overview of the Mathias criteria to demonstrate occupational causation/aggravation, (2) a description of which Mathias criteria were met and physician justification, (3) acknowledgment that because at least 4 of the 7 criteria were met, there was a reasonable degree of medical certainty for OCD, and (4) specific instructions regarding treatment, preventative measures, and rehabilitation, as well as prognosis and projected recovery times for the worker(s). Logical conclusions should be drawn, and a note should be made on the physician's availability to answer any further questions should they arise.

PROGNOSIS

The prognosis of OCD depends on many factors. Removal of the allergen and replacement with a different product is key to worker improvement, if possible; however, often this cannot be achieved owing to the nature of the work causing disease. Unfortunately, many studies have shown that contact dermatitis persists when jobs are kept. In addition, studies have shown that the duration of symptoms before diagnosis is correlated with a poorer prognosis and recalcitrant disease. Intensive treatment may still be of use in these situations; in a recent study by Skudlik and colleagues[36] involving 1164 workers in high-risk professions, the efficacy of a 6-week, intensive treatment period termed tertiary individual prevention was evaluated. The program required in-patient and out-patient treatments by local dermatologists, coupled with individual motivation and workplace support. Sixty-six percent of the workers were able to successfully remain in their professions, and results were durable. Although it may be difficult to complete the intensive regimen, it is worth making employers and employees aware of this treatment plan if the OCD is severe and recalcitrant. Additionally, lifestyle factors may be of major importance influencing occupational dermatitis. Olesen and colleagues[16] reported that tobacco smoking and high stress levels had an inverse relationship to healing occupational hand dermatitis, whereas high levels of exercise was significantly related to healing, as well as change of profession, predictably. Age, sex, AD history, and education were also found in previous studies to have an impact on OCD.[24]

Generally, factors leading to improved prognosis involve removal and avoidance of the causative agent, worker education, and proper treatment. For the dermatologist, being readily available and establishing worker relationships are also central.

DISCLOSURE

The authors have nothing to disclose.

REFERENCES

1. Sasseville D. Occupational contact dermatitis. Allergy Asthma Clin Immunol 2008;4(2):59.
2. Luckhaupt SE, Dahlhamer JM, Ward BW, et al. Prevalence of dermatitis in the working population, United States, 2010 National Health Interview Survey. Am J Ind Med 2013;56(6):625–34.
3. Wiszniewska M, Walusiak-Skorupa J. Recent trends in occupational contact dermatitis. Curr Allergy Asthma Rep 2015;15(7). https://doi.org/10.1007/s11882-015-0543-z.
4. Holness DL. Health care services use by workers with work-related contact dermatitis. Dermatitis 2004;15(1):18–24. Available at: http://www.ncbi.nlm.nih.gov/pubmed/15573644. Accessed August 29, 2019.
5. Lampel HP, Atwater AR. Patch testing tools of the trade: use of immunosuppressants and antihistamines during patch testing. J Dermatol Nurses Assoc 2016;8(3):209–11.
6. Grob JJ, Castelain M, Richard MA, et al. Antiinflammatory properties of cetirizine in a human contact dermatitis model. clinical evaluation of patch tests is not hampered by antihistamines. Acta Derm Venereol 1998;78(3):194–7.
7. Halling-Overgaard AS, Kezic S, Jakasa I, et al. Skin absorption through atopic dermatitis skin: a systematic review. Br J Dermatol 2017. https://doi.org/10.1111/bjd.15065.
8. Mathias CGT. Periodic synopsis. Occupational dermatoses. J Am Acad Dermatol 1988;19. https://doi.org/10.1016/S0190-9622(98)80005-4.
9. Ingber A, Merims S. The validity of the Mathias criteria for establishing occupational causation and aggravation of contact dermatitis. Contact Dermatitis 2004;51(1):9–12.

10. Handa S, De D, Mahajan R. Airborne contact dermatitis-current perspectives in etiopathogenesis and management. Indian J Dermatol 2011;56(6):700–6.

11. Bourke J, Coulson I, English J. Guidelines for the management of contact dermatitis: an update. Br J Dermatol 2009;160(5):946–54.

12. Uyesugi BA, Sheehan MP. Patch testing pearls. Clin Rev Allergy Immunol 2019;56(1):110–8.

13. Chaudhry HM, Drage LA, El-Azhary RA, et al. Delayed patch-test reading after 5 days: an update from the Mayo Clinic Contact Dermatitis Group. Dermatitis 2017;28(4):253–60.

14. de Groot AC, Liem DH, Nater JP, et al. Patch tests with fragrance materials and preservatives. Contact Dermatitis 1985;12(2):87–92.

15. Mowad CM, Anderson B, Scheinman P, et al. Allergic contact dermatitis Patient management and education. J Am Acad Dermatol 2016;74(6):1043–54.

16. Olesen CM, Agner T, Ebbehøj NE, et al. Factors influencing prognosis for occupational hand eczema: new trends. Br J Dermatol 2019. https://doi.org/10.1111/bjd.17870.

17. Brown TP. Strategies for prevention: occupational contact. Occup Med (Chic Ill) 2004;54(7):450–7.

18. Schnetz E, Diepgen TL, Elsner P, et al. Multicentre study for the development of an in vivo model to evaluate the influence of topical formulations on irritation. Contact Dermatitis 2000;42(6):336–43.

19. Berndt U, Wigger-Alberti W, Gabard B, et al. Efficacy of a barrier cream and its vehicle as protective measures against occupational irritant contact dermatitis. Contact Dermatitis 2000;42(2):77–80.

20. Goh CL, Gan SL. Efficacies of a barrier cream and an afterwork emollient cream against cutting fluid dermatitis in metalworkers: a prospective study. Contact Dermatitis 1994;31(3):176–80.

21. Elsner P. Skin protection in the prevention of skin diseases. Curr Probl Dermatol 2007;34:1–10.

22. Winker R, Salameh B, Stolkovich S, et al. Effectiveness of skin protection creams in the prevention of occupational dermatitis: results of a randomized, controlled trial. Int Arch Occup Environ Health 2009;82(5):653–62.

23. Saary J, Qureshi R, Palda V, et al. A systematic review of contact dermatitis treatment and prevention. J Am Acad Dermatol 2005;53(5):845.e1–13.

24. Clark SC, Zirwas MJ. Management of occupational dermatitis. Dermatol Clin 2009;27(3):365–83.

25. Williams C, Wilkinson SM, McShane P, et al. A double-blind, randomized study to assess the effectiveness of different moisturizers in preventing dermatitis induced by hand washing to simulate healthcare use. Br J Dermatol 2010;162(5):1088–92.

26. Wortzman MS, Scott RA, Wong PS, et al. Soap and detergent bar rinsability. J Soc Cosmet Chem 1986;37:89–97.

27. Brazzini B, Pimpinelli N. New and established topical corticosteroids in dermatology: clinical pharmacology and therapeutic use. Am J Clin Dermatol 2002;3(1):47–58.

28. Hachem JP, De Paepe K, Vanpée E, et al. Efficacy of topical corticosteroids in nickel-induced contact allergy. Clin Exp Dermatol 2002;27(1):47–50. Available at: http://www.ncbi.nlm.nih.gov/pubmed/11952670. Accessed August 19, 2019.

29. Levin C, Zhai H, Bashir S, et al. Efficacy of corticosteroids in acute experimental irritant contact dermatitis? Skin Res Technol 2001;7(4):214–8. Available at: http://www.ncbi.nlm.nih.gov/pubmed/11737815. Accessed August 19, 2019.

30. Özgüç Çömlek F, Örüm S, Aydın S, et al. Exogenous Cushing syndrome due to misuse of potent topical steroid. Pediatr Dermatol 2018;35(2):e121–3.

31. Veien NK, Larsen PØ, Thestrup-Pedersen K, et al. Long-term, intermittent treatment of chronic hand eczema with mometasone furoate. Br J Dermatol 1999;140(5):882–6.

32. Matura M, Goossens A, Matura M. Contact allergy to corticosteroids. Allergy 2000;55(8):698–704.

33. Isaksson M. Corticosteroid contact allergy - The importance of late readings and testing with corticosteroids used by the patients. Contact Dermatitis 2007;56(1):56–7.

34. Katsarou A, Makris M, Papagiannaki K, et al. Tacrolimus 0.1% vs mometasone furoate topical treatment in allergic contact hand eczema: a prospective randomized clinical study. Eur J Dermatol 2012;22(2):192–6.

35. Owen JL, Vakharia PP, Silverberg JI. The role and diagnosis of allergic contact dermatitis in patients with atopic dermatitis. Am J Clin Dermatol 2018;19(3):293–302.

36. Skudlik C, Wulfhorst B, Gediga G, et al. Tertiary individual prevention of occupational skin diseases: a decade's experience with recalcitrant occupational dermatitis. Int Arch Occup Environ Health 2008;81(8):1059–64.

Occupational Contact Dermatitis
Common Occupational Allergens

Christopher Chu, MD, James G. Marks Jr, MD, Alexandra Flamm, MD*

KEYWORDS

- Occupational skin disease • Contact dermatitis • Allergens • Patch testing

KEY POINTS

- Contact dermatitis, both irritant and allergic, accounts for the majority of occupational skin disease.
- Occupations at high risk for occupational allergic contact dermatitis include agricultural workers, construction workers, health care workers, hairdressers, mechanics, and machinists.
- Understanding allergen exposures in high-risk occupations can help to guide the history and physical examination, and help clinicians to choose allergens for patch testing.

INTRODUCTION

The prevalence of occupational contact dermatitis has been estimated to be anywhere between 6.7% and 10.6%.[1] Contact dermatitis, both allergic and irritant, accounts for about 80% of all causes of occupational skin disease.[2] When suspecting occupational allergic contact dermatitis (ACD), a general understanding of the patients' daily work as well as their exposures may help to narrow down potential culprits. Oftentimes, the standard patch test tray may need to be expanded and individuals exposed to workplace contact allergens may need to undergo patch testing to special series of allergens relevant to their occupations.

The occupations at highest risk for skin disease include nurses and other health care professionals, precision workers in metals and related materials, hairdressers and beauticians, butchers and cooks, and tool makers and related trade workers (**Box 1**).[3] Furthermore, thousands of different products may result in occupational contact dermatitis. Overall, formaldehyde, carba mix, thiuram mix, epoxy resin, and nickel are the most common patch test allergens associated with occupational ACD.[4,5] This article reviews common occupations at high risk for occupational contact dermatitis and their potential relevant allergens.

AGRICULTURAL WORKERS

Agricultural workers perform a variety of jobs and are exposed to a wide variety of chemical, biologic, and physical hazards. This exposure includes growth of crops that require preparing the soil for planting, fertilizing, cultivating, and harvesting. They clean and repair farm equipment, and livestock contact is often seen. Their chemical exposures include veterinary medications, feed additives, and pesticides. Because currently farming is extremely specialized, knowing the type of agricultural work performed is vital for ascertaining the possible source for a suspected occupationally induced ACD (**Table 1**).

In 2006, the United States Bureau of Labor Statistics reported that the incidence of skin disease was 16.5 per 10,000 workers employed in crop production in 2005. A study of 304 farmers in North Carolina found that 12.2% of farmers had contact dermatitis, although it was unclear whether these were irritant or allergen related.[6] Risk factors identified in this subset of farmworkers included young age, pesticide exposure, and poor housing conditions, all of which may contribute to poor hygiene practices after work.[6]

In a Polish study, 87 of 101 farmers who reported occupational dermatoses were diagnosed

Department of Dermatology, Penn State Hershey, 500 University Drive, Hershey, PA 17033, USA
* Corresponding author.
E-mail address: aflamm@pennstatehealth.psu.edu

Dermatol Clin 38 (2020) 339–349
https://doi.org/10.1016/j.det.2020.02.002
0733-8635/20/© 2020 Elsevier Inc. All rights reserved.

Agricultural workers

Construction workers

Health care workers (nurses, dentists)

Florists

Hairdressers

Housekeeping personnel

Mechanics

Machinists

Food service workers

with ACD.[7] The most common chemical allergens were metals, most commonly chromium, cobalt, and nickel; chemical allergens including pesticides like malathion; and rubber additives such as thiuram.[7]

Although culprit allergens such as metals are more ubiquitous, pesticides are a unique exposure of agricultural workers. In addition to the active ingredients in pesticides, inactive substances such as emulsifiers, surfactants, or biocides may cause irritation or allergic reactions. Although pesticide contact dermatitis is most likely quite common, it remains underreported because the implicated pesticides vary across regions and according to crop patterns. In an Indian study, 33.3% of patients showed a positive patch test to pesticide ingredients, most commonly thiuram mix, propiconazole, mercaptobenzothiazole, and formaldehyde. Although thiuram mix is often seen in the context of rubber glove use, in agricultural workers thiuram mix is also used in pesticides as a fungicide.[8] In affected patients, uncovered areas were primarily involved, suggesting the major predisposing factor for pesticide dermatitis continues to be direct or airborne contact with the pesticide. Personal protective equipment, gloves,

and avoiding direct skin contact are the most important preventative measures. Despite the prevalence of ACD to pesticides in agricultural workers, no standardized pesticide patch test series is currently available.

Agricultural work has become increasingly more specialized. It is imperative to clarify the type of work the specific patient in question is performing. Although some exposures may be more common in all farmers such as metals, and thiuram mix from exposure to rubber gloves, pesticide and animal exposure may be unique to the patient's line of work.

CONSTRUCTION WORKERS

Construction workers encompass a broad spectrum of occupations including carpenters, masons, electricians, painters, and plumbers. On some construction sites workers do several of these tasks. The exposure varies depending on the work performed by the worker (**Table 2**).

Carpenters are involved in rough and finished woodworking, such as installing doors and windows, and molding. Most cases of occupationally induced ACD from wood dust is due to tropical woods such as teak; ACD from the nontropical wood used most commonly by carpenters is rare.[9]

Masons and cement workers are at the greatest risk for ACD in the construction industry. The most common cause is the water-soluble hexavalent chromate in cement. Specifically, patch tested brick layers are much more likely to be positive to potassium dichromate, rubber, and cobalt than nonconstruction workers. The sensitization to potassium dichromate directly comes from contact with cement, which often have varying concentrations of chromate. Sensitization to rubber

Table 1
Common occupational allergens in agricultural workers

Exposure	Allergen(s)
Metals	Nickel
	Chromium
	Cobalt
Pesticides ingredients[a]	Malathion
	Propiconazole
	Mercaptobenzothiazole
	Formaldehyde
Rubber additives	Thiuram mix

[a] Pesticide ingredients may vary depending on the region.

Table 2
Common occupational allergens in construction workers

Profession	Allergen
Carpenters	Tropical woods
Cement workers	Potassium dichromate
Electricians	Colophony
Painters	MCI/MI
	Epoxy resin
	Formaldehyde
	Quaternium-15
Plumbers	Acrylates
	Epoxy resin

Abbreviation: MCI/MI, methylchloroisothiazolinone/methylisothiazolinone.

is due to use of rubber gloves, the main personal protective equipment used by construction workers. Cobalt is a cosensitizer with chromium, which may explain the high rates of sensitization in this group.[10,11]

Electricians install various electrical fixtures such as lights and wire buildings. They use soldering fluxes that contain colophony (also known as rosin) to join wires together, which can cause occupational ACD.[12]

Painters are responsible for covering holes and cracks with fillers and sanding surfaces before painting. Historically, the most frequent cause of ACD in painters was turpentine, but these have since been replaced by cheaper substitutes such as petroleum-based white spirits.[13] Painters are more likely to be sensitized to methylchloroisothiazolinone/methylisothiazolinone (MCI/MI), epoxy resin, formaldehyde, and quaternium-15.[14] MCI/MI is currently found in paint, and has also been found in other studies to be a common cause of occupational contact dermatitis in painters.[15] Airborne allergies to MI resulting in ACD and asthma in painters has also been published, suggesting a potential for airborne sensitivity.[16] Epoxy resins, found as a binding material in paint, is another common cause of occupational contact dermatitis in painters.[14,17] Formaldehyde is found in paint in small amounts, and may also cause sensitization in painters. Although quaternium-15, a formaldehyde-releaser, is not normally found in paint, cross-reactions between patients sensitized to formaldehyde and formaldehyde releasers are common.

Plumbers may become allergic to the methacrylates found in glues, sealants, and adhesives.[18] Occupational ACD to acrylates from the coating material used on pipes has also been reported.[19] Plumbers have also been reported to have occupational ACD to diethylenetriamine in epoxy resins.[20]

HEALTH CARE WORKERS INCLUDING DENTAL WORKERS

Health care workers such as physicians, nurses, and health aides, as well as dentists and dental hygienists, have a high rate of occupational skin disease, with 1 report from a 1993 Bureau of Labor Statistics survey reporting the highest number of occupational contact dermatitis in the health service industry.[21] In another study evaluating the occupation of patients diagnosed with occupational dermatitis, registered nurses were the most frequent occupation affected.[22] Health care workers are exposed to numerous chemicals, such as soaps, antiseptics, fragrances, or glove ingredients. Many of these agents can cause both irritant contact dermatitis (ICD) and ACD (**Table 3**).

Table 3
Common occupational allergens in health care workers

Exposure	Allergen
Rubber accelerators	Thiuram mix
	Carba mix
	Zinc diethyldithiocarbamate
Preservatives/ Disinfectants	Glutaraldehyde
	Cocamide DEA
	Quaternium-15
	Benzalkonium
Adhesives	Colophonium
Misc.	Acrylates

In a study by the North American Contact Dermatitis Group (NACDG), more than 1255 health care workers patch tested were compared with a total group of 15,896 non-health care workers patch tested. Female sex and hand involvement were significantly more common among health care workers, although this may be a reflection of the female predominance in some areas of health care. Health care workers were significantly more likely to have reactions to thiuram mix, carba mix, glutaraldehyde, cocamide diethanolamine (DEA), and chloroxylenol.

The high frequency of hand dermatitis likely correlates with the high frequency of ACD to the rubber accelerators thiuram mix and carba mix found in gloves. This factor, coupled with frequent hand washing, increases the risk of developing an ACD to these chemicals. Glutaraldehyde is a biocide commonly used in cold-sterilizing buffered solutions for disinfecting delicate medical instruments. It is also found in preservatives and disinfectants and more than one-half of occupation-related reactions to glutaraldehyde occurred in health care workers working in dentistry (**Fig. 1**). DEA is a surfactant found in cleansers and shampoos, and all reactions to DEA were found in health care workers with direct patient interaction, who generally wash hands between patient care tasks. Chloroxylenol is a phenol antiseptic used for its antiseptic properties in hand washes and is also found in preservatives in medicaments, electrocardiography paste, and over-the-counter products.[23] Eleven patients also reacted to methylmethacrylates, and 8 of these patients worked in dentistry. The relevance of this is discussed elsewhere in this article.

Other studies have also noted that health care workers with occupational ACD were more likely to be female and to have hand dermatitis. Other allergens that were more commonly noted in health care worker included quaternium-15, thimerosal, benzalkonium chloride, potassium dichromate,

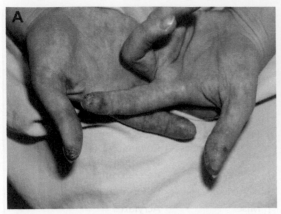 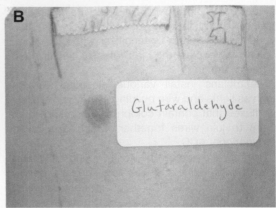

Fig. 1. (A) A medical worker with dermatitis of the fingertips. (B) The patient subsequently patch tested positive to glutaraldehyde, a biocide. (*Courtesy of* J. G. Marks Jr., MD, Hershey, PA.)

MCI/MI, colophonium, 2-bromo-2-nitropropane-1,3-diol, and zinc diethyldithiocarbmate.[24,25]

Quaternium-15 is a formaldehyde-releasing preservative used in many cosmetics and industrial substances, such as liquid soaps, moisturizers, and cleaning supplies. Thimerosal, an organic mercury compound, is used as a preservative in vaccines, and although it could be explained by the increased rate of vaccination among this group, it is also a very common patch test positive allergen, whose relevance to active dermatitis is rarely found. Benzalkonium chloride is widely used in hand sanitizers, especially alcohol-free hand sanitizers, and as disinfectants for floors and surgical equipment.[24]

Patients become sensitized to potassium dichromate largely through the contact with chrome-tanned leather, and it is unclear why nurses had an increased rate of sensitization. Colophonium is found in adhesive plasters, bandages, or hydrocolloid dressings. MCI/MI is a preservative often found in skin care products such as hand or barrier creams and liquid soaps. Zinc diethyldithiocarbamate (ZDEC) is another rubber accelerator similar to thiuram.[25] It has also been reported that health care workers are more likely to have allergic contact urticaria to latex.[26]

The occupational allergen spectrum in health care workers, although broad, has not changed significantly in the past decade. Health care workers with occupational contact dermatitis are most likely to have hand dermatitis and are more likely to be female. The main ingredients that continue to cause occupational dermatitis in health care workers include rubber accelerators such as thiuram mix, carba mix, and ZDEC. Other causes are disinfectants, surfactants, or preservatives found in skin care products such as soaps and sterilizing solutions, such as glutaraldehyde, cocamide DEA, quaternium-15, and benzalkonium. An

increase in ACD to colophonium, which is often found in adhesives has also been noted.

DENTAL WORKERS

Dentists and dental personnel, similar to health care personnel, have a high risk of occupational contact dermatitis owing to frequent hand washing, increased use of latex gloves, and contact with disinfectants and local anesthetics. The prevalence of occupational contact dermatitis in dental personnel ranges between 15% and 33%.[27] Although sensitivities to biocides such as glutaraldehyde and latex have been historically common in dental personnel, ACD to glutaraldehyde has markedly decreased with the substitution of nonglutaraldehydes, such as chlorine dioxide solutions or ortho-phthaladehyde. Dental personnel, however, do have a unique exposure to metals and acrylic monomers also known as methacrylates and acrylates (**Fig. 2**). In dentistry, acrylics are used to make bridges and crowns, dentures and other prostheses, and for the repair of fractured prostheses.[28] Most studies have demonstrated consistently the common culprit of methacrylates, with percentages ranging from 6.1% to 22.0%.[29-31] The rate of occupational ACD to metals has had conflicting evidence, with some sources quoting nickel allergy rates as high as 37%, and other studies demonstrating no increased sensitivity to metals.[29,30]

Interestingly, some studies have noted dental technicians did not have an increased frequency of sensitization to rubber chemicals, despite presumed frequent use of protective gloves. This is likely owing to the recommendation that nitrile gloves be worn for no longer than 10 minutes to protect against acrylate/methacrylate penetration.[30]

Because contact with methacrylates causing occupational ACD is mostly on the hands, gloves

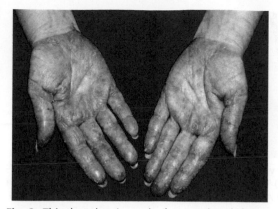

Fig. 2. This dental assistant had severe hand dermatitis for 2 years. Patch test subsequently tested positive for glutaraldehyde and acrylates, both common culprits for occupational ACD in dental workers. (*Courtesy of* J. G. Marks Jr., MD, Hershey, PA.)

are of the utmost importance. The most preferred combination of hand protection against acrylates/methacrylates is wearing a polyethylene glove underneath a nitrile glove.[30,32]

FLORISTS

Florists design and arrange floral displays by cutting, clipping, and breaking flowers and greenery. A pocketknife is often used to cut the stems, which can cause small cuts of the thumb. Florists use foam bases, floral preservatives, wire pins, tape, ribbons, and spray paint. They may also be responsible for watering, trimming, and repotting live plants.

In 1 review, the prevalence of occupational ACD in a large US floral company was found to be 26%.[13,33] The most frequent positive patch test was to tuliposide A, the allergen in both the *Alstroemeria* and *Liliacea* species (**Table 4**).

The frequency of occupational ACD to tulips and its allergen tuliposide A is so common that the term tulip finger has been used to describe an erythematous, pruritic, scaling dermatitis that affects the forefingers and thumb of tulip bulb workers (**Fig. 3**).[34] For tuliposide A, nitrile gloves have been found to provide better protection than vinyl gloves.[35]

Occupational ACD to sesquiterpene lactones in florists has also been reported.[36,37] Sesquiterpene lactones are important allergens in the Compositae, Umbelliferae, and Magnoliaceae families. The compositae family encompasses a number of popular plants, including dandelions, arnica, and chrysanthemum. Umbelliferae includes such plants as celery, parsley, and carrots. If a compositae allergy is suspected, no single sesquiterpene lactone or mix is adequate to screen for a compositae allergy, so it is recommended that the portion of the specific chrysanthemum plant handled by a florist be tested.[38]

Another common plant allergen handled by florists that causes ACD is the English primrose, *Primula obconica*. This popular household plant can cause dermatitis in housewives and patch testing is done with synthetic primin (**Fig. 4**).[39]

Of note, the presence of allergens is not uniform within sensitizing floral species. A particular species may have hundreds of varieties of cultivars that do not possess the same amount of allergens. Even within a single plant, the amount of allergens varies among the bulb, leaf, petal, and stem and according the plant's stage of growth.[40]

ICD is also common in florists, owing to repeated wet work and minor trauma from thorns, stems, wires, and irritating sap. Examples of potent irritant plants include Euphorbia (Spurge), Narcissus, and Dieffenbachia (dumb cane).[13]

HAIRDRESSERS

Hairdressers clean, condition, cut, wave, style, and color hair. They have a high risk of ICD from frequent shampooing, which leads to impaired skin barrier and likely heightened absorption of allergenic compounds, causing increased rates of ACD (**Table 5**). Some of the common allergens include nickel in their instruments, rubber chemicals in gloves, p-phenylenediamine in permanent hair colors, glyceryl monothioglycolate (GMTG) in permanent hair waving solutions, and ammonium persulfate in hair bleach (**Fig. 5**).[41–45] Of note, GMTG avoidance is difficult because it typically contaminates the work surfaces of the shop.[41] Complete withdrawal of GMTG from some countries resulted in a decrease in the prevalence of GMTG allergy.[42]

In general, most studies have shown the risk of ACD is higher than ICD in this population.[41,43] The most common site of involvement was the hand.[43]

Other positive allergens that have been noted in this population include 2-hydroxyethyl methacrylate and quaternium-15. The compound 2-hydroxyethyl methacrylate is a common acrylate

Table 4
Common occupational allergens in florist

Exposure	Allergen
Alstroemeria (Peruvian Lily) Liliacea (Tulips)	Tuliposide A
Compositae (eg, Chrysanthemum)	Sesquiterpene Lactones
Primrose	Primin

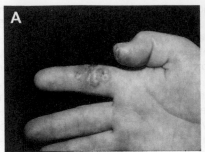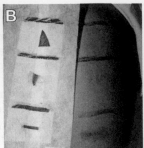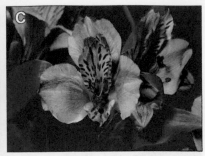

Fig. 3. (*A*) This florist demonstrates classic "tulip fingers," with erythematous, pruritic, scaling dermatitis that affects the forefingers and thumb of tulip bulb workers. (*B*) This patient was subsequently found to have positive patch testing to the stem of the Peruvian Lily, part of the Alstromeria family. (*C*) Peruvian Lily. (*Courtesy of* J. G. Marks Jr., MD, Hershey, PA.)

sensitizer found in artificial nail products and quaternium-15 is found in many makeups, lotions, and other cosmetics. Of note, however, this finding was reported in a population that included hairdressers and cosmetologists, which could explain the prevalence of these allergens in this study. Other studies have also found frequent positivity to toluene-2,5-diamine, another ingredient of hair dyes.[44,45]

Hairdressers are at particularly high risk for occupational contact dermatitis owing to the exposure to numerous chemicals and tools in combination. Specifically, the ammonium thioglycolate can cause release of nickel from the tools, leading to a higher frequency of nickel ACD.[46] Additionally, because many hairdressers may become sensitized to rubber gloves and because GMTG penetrates rubber gloves more readily, hairdressers should wear vinyl or nitrile gloves.

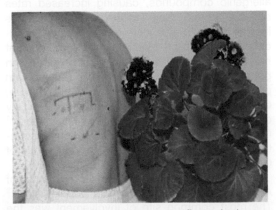

Fig. 4. This patient, who was not a florist, had severe hand and facial dermatitis and subsequently tested positive to primin, the allergen in primrose. Her husband had given her primroses 3 months before the onset of her dermatitis. (*Courtesy of* J. G. Marks Jr., MD, Hershey, PA.)

HOUSEKEEPING PERSONNEL

Housekeeping personnel can include anyone working at home or in any business place. They frequently have exposure to numerous cleaning and disinfectant chemicals. As with other employees in wet work occupations, such as health care workers and food industry workers, cleaners are prone to sensitization owing to daily skin contact with different cleaners and surface disinfectants (**Table 6**).

Most studies have found that although there is a high frequency of occupational skin disease, housekeeping personnel are largely affected by ICD as opposed to ACD.[47,48] However, the rates of ACD have been reported to be as high as 38% in some studies, so this is overall variable.[49] The most common allergens noted include formaldehyde, glutaraldehyde, chloramine, nickel, and rubber chemicals and accelerators, such as thiurams, ZDEC, and mercaptobenzothiazole.[47–49]

Other relevant allergens found in housekeeping personnel included benzalkonium chloride, glyoxal, and glutaraldehyde, which are all disinfectants.[49] The most common causes of occupational ACD in housekeeping personnel parallel those seen in the health care worker. Because protective gloves are used over long periods of time during working hours and there is prolonged skin contact with

Table 5
Common occupational allergens in hairdressers

Exposure	Allergen
Permanent hair waving solutions	GMTG
Hair bleaching products	Ammonium persulfate
Hair dyes	p-Phenylenediamine
Hairdresser tools	Nickel

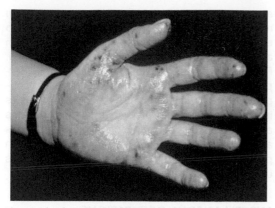

Fig. 5. This hairdresser had severe hand dermatitis for 2 years. She patch tested positive to glyceryl thioglycolate, which is used in acidic permanent wave solutions. A switch to alkaline perms improved, but did not resolve, her hand dermatitis. (*Courtesy of* J. G. Marks Jr., MD, Hershey, PA.)

rubber chemicals, there are high rates of positivity to rubber accelerators such as thiurams, ZDEC, and mercaptobenzothiazole. One recommendation is to switch to thick, reusable, loose-fitting, cotton-lined gloves. Not only do these kinds of gloves prevents contact with aggressive cleaning products and water, they show lower amounts of rubber chemical residues than single use medical gloves.[50] However, many cleaners continue to use only single-use medical gloves, which contain higher amounts of rubber chemical residues and lead to intensive skin contact with allergens owing to their tight fit.

MECHANICS

Mechanics repair cars, trucks, and buses. They do routine maintenance such as lubrication, oil changes, and tire rotations and are exposed to many irritants and allergens, especially on the hands. They are exposed to a variety of irritating fuels, cleansers, and solvents and often clean

themselves with gasoline and abrasive soaps (**Table 7**).

In a Swedish study, 15% of mechanics surveyed reported hand eczema. The most common diagnosis was ICD, although 19% of patients had ACD, most frequently to thimerosal, nickel, and colophony. However, although thimerosal was prevalent, it was no more prevalent than in the general population and therefore not deemed clinically relevant. Nickel-plated tools are very common and are most likely the source of occupationally relevant nickel-related ACD. Like many of the other professions at high risk for occupational ACD, mechanics are exposed to solvents and irritants that can increase their likelihood of becoming sensitized to allergens like nickel.[51]

The NACDG analyzed 691 mechanics/repairers with ACD and found that hand dermatitis was the most common presentation, and carba mix, thiuram mix, and MCI/MI were the most common clinically relevant allergens. As discussed elsewhere in this article, carba mix and thiuram mix are common rubber accelerators, and the protective gloves used by many mechanics contain additives from the rubber manufacturing process. MCI/MI are common allergens found in cleansers, hand soaps, and other skin care products. Waterless hand cleansers marketed to mechanics are a frequent source of ACD caused by MCI/MI. Metals and preservatives were common allergens found in electrical and electronic equipment mechanics/repairers.[52] Other common allergens noted in studies of this population included epoxy resin, potassium dichromate, and p-phenylenediamine, although the latter may be of unclear relevance.[53]

PRODUCTION WORKERS: MACHINISTS AND PRINTING MACHINE OPERATORS

Production workers may be involved in multiple steps needed to produce a final metal product. A classic example of a production worker is a machinist, who is responsible for operating metal cutting machines. Other fields considered production workers include printing machine operators, who may be responsible for loading a printing

Table 6
Common occupational allergens in housekeeping personnel

Exposure	Allergen
Disinfectants	Benzalkonium chloride Glyoxal Glutaraldehyde Chloramine
Rubber accelerators	Thiuram mix ZDEC Mercaptobenzothiazole
Preservatives	Formaldehyde

Table 7
Common occupational allergens in mechanics

Exposure	Allergen
Metals	Nickel Potassium dichromate
Rubber accelerators	Thiuram mix Carba mix
Preservatives	MCI/MI

press with stock and ink and removing printed materials (**Table 8**).

Metalworking fluids are a universal requirement in the job of a machinist, because the fluid is required to cool and lubricate the machines. These fluids are a large source of the occupational ACD found in machinists. In a Finnish study, the most common allergens among machinists were antimicrobials such as formaldehyde. Other common causes included ethanolamines and colophony, which are emulsifiers used in metalworking fluids.[54]

The NACDG reviewed 2732 production workers and found that the most common causes of occupational ACD were epoxy, thiuram mix, carba mix, formaldehyde, and cobalt. Epoxy adhesives are used for manufacturing of aircrafts, vehicles, hockey sticks, and other goods, which require high-strength bonds. In 1 study of occupational contact dermatitis caused by epoxy chemicals, more than one-half of the 209 cases were patients who worked in industrial trades, such as aircraft production, manufacturing of electric machines, and wiring.[55] Thiuram mix and carba mix are rubber accelerators used in the production of the thin natural rubber latex gloves or synthetic nitrile gloves that production workers wear to allow for dexterity. Formaldehyde is a biocide used in many metalworking fluids and cutting oils, and in a study of patients with formaldehyde allergy, metalworkers comprised the greatest proportion of occupational sensitization.[56] Finally, given that their primary job is to interact with metals, there is no surprise that metal is a commonly noted allergen. Even the coatings, paints, and adhesives used in metalworking may contain cobalt or other metals to hasten the drying process.[57]

Printing machine operators share similar exposures to machinists, but also note ACD owing to components of ink. In a study of printing machine operators by the NACDG, cobalt, carba mix, thiuram mix, and formaldehyde were the most common causes of occupation-related ACD. As described elsewhere in this article, glove use likely account to the positivity to carba mix and thiuram mix; however, cobalt ACD is likely attributed to exposure to inks and coatings, because it is often added to catalyze the oxidation and drying of inks. Formaldehyde is similarly used in many letterpresses and inks. Less common causes of occupational ACD in printing machine operators include acrylates and propylene glycol. Acrylates are components of many ultraviolet-cured inks and printing plates. Propylene glycol is found in printing press fountain solution and the cleansers used to clean the printing press.[58]

MISCELLANEOUS OCCUPATIONS
Food Service Workers

Food service workers are also at high risk of occupational skin disease, owing to their high rates of wet work. The most common sensitivities were nickel sulfate, thiuram mix, carba mix, formaldehyde, and compositae mix.[59,60] Of note, there was no increase in sensitization to fragrance mix and balsam of Peru, which is often found in spices, foods, and flavoring agents. Although nickel sulfate is a common allergen overall, the rates seemed to be higher in the food processing industry, possibly attributable to the increased exposure to steel cooking instruments. Thiuram mix and carba mix, also found in other industries in which employees frequently wear gloves, is more common in food workers. The high rate of formaldehyde positivity is most likely due to the increased use of cleansers and handwashing.[59] Compositae mix positivity may be explained by the increase contact with certain vegetables that are in the family, such as chicory and iceberg lettuce.

Of note, contact urticaria does have a higher prevalence in food service workers compared with non-food service workers. A variety of proteins and chemicals are known to cause contact urticaria, and food-related skin prick testing may be helpful in evaluating food service workers with hand dermatitis.[60]

Musicians

Occupational skin disease in musicians is most often due to callosities such as fiddler's neck, as opposed to ACD. Violinists and violists reported the most ACD. The most common allergens were to nickel and colophonium, which is commonly used by string players to wax their strings to increase the attrition between the bow and the strings. Nickel sensitization may be due to the overall prevalence of nickel allergy in the general population, as opposed to an occupational exposure.[61,62] Other reported allergens in the literature

Table 8
Common occupational allergens in production workers

Exposure	Allergen
Adhesives	Epoxy resin Colophony
Rubber accelerators	Thiuram mix Carba mix
Metals	Nickel Cobalt
Preservatives	Formaldehyde

in musicians include propolis from violin varnishes and rosewoods in a Basque wind instrument.[63,64]

Office Workers

Office personnel are employed predominantly in managerial and clerical positions. Office workers are not typically at high risk for occupationally related ACD owing to their limited exposure to harsh chemicals. However, it is worth noting that there seems to be potential for ACD owing to paper, and there has been a case report describing colophony positivity owing to extracts from newspaper.[65]

SUMMARY

There are numerous occupations at high risk for ACD, and even more possible culprits. Although obtaining the occupation is key as an initial step in the evaluation of occupational ACD, knowing the common allergens may help to guide the history and physical examination, as well as help the astute clinician to choose allergens for patch testing.

DISCLOSURE

The authors have nothing to disclose.

REFERENCES

1. Mostosi C, Simonart T. Effectiveness of barrier creams against irritant contact dermatitis. Dermatology 2016;232(3):353–62.
2. Belsito DV. Occupational contact dermatitis: etiology, prevalence, and resultant impairment/disability. J Am Acad Dermatol 2005;53(2):303–13.
3. Bensefa-Colas L, Telle-Lamberton M, Paris C, et al. Occupational allergic contact dermatitis and major allergens in France: temporal trends for the period 2001-2010. Br J Dermatol 2014;171(6):1375–85.
4. Wiszniewska M, Walusiak-Skorupa J. Recent trends in occupational contact dermatitis. Curr Allergy Asthma Rep 2015;15(7). https://doi.org/10.1007/s11882-015-0543-z.
5. Adisesh A, Robinson E, Nicholson PJ, et al. U.K. standards of care for occupational contact dermatitis and occupational contact urticaria. Br J Dermatol 2013;168(6):1167–75.
6. Arcury TA, Feldman SR, Schulz MR, et al. Diagnosed skin diseases among migrant farmworkers in North Carolina: prevalence and risk factors. J Agric Saf Health 2007;13(4):407–18.
7. Spiewak R. Occupational dermatoses among Polish private farmers, 1991-1999. Am J Ind Med 2003; 43(6):647–55.
8. Sharma A, Mahajan VK, Mehta KS, et al. Pesticide contact dermatitis in agricultural workers of Himachal Pradesh (India). Contact Dermatitis 2018;79(4):213–7.
9. Estlander T, Jolanki R, Alanko K, et al. Occupational allergic contact dermatitis caused by wood dusts. Contact Dermatitis 2001;44(4):213–7.
10. Lazzarini R, Duarte IAG, Sumita JM, et al. Dermatite alérgica de contato entre pedreiros, num serviço não especializado em dermatoses ocupacionais. An Bras Dermatol 2012;87(4):567–71.
11. Uter W, Rühl R, Pfahlberg A, et al. Contact allergy in construction workers: results of a multifactorial analysis. Ann Occup Hyg 2004;48(1):21–7.
12. Toby Mathias CG, Adams RM. Allergic contact dermatitis from rosin used as soldering flux. J Am Acad Dermatol 1984;10(3):454–6.
13. Marks JG, Anderson BE, DeLeo VA. Contact and occupational dermatology. 4th edition. Jaypee Brothers Medical; 2016.
14. Mose AP, Lundov MD, Zachariae C, et al. Occupational contact dermatitis in painters - an analysis of patch test data from the Danish Contact Dermatitis Group. Contact Dermatitis 2012;67(5):293–7.
15. Fischer T, Bohlin S, Edling C, et al. Skin disease and contact sensitivity in house painters using water-based paints, glues and putties. Contact Dermatitis 1995;32(1):39–45.
16. Lundov MD, Mosbech H, Thyssen JP, et al. Two cases of airborne allergic contact dermatitis caused by methylisothiazolinone in paint. Contact Dermatitis 2011. https://doi.org/10.1111/j.1600-0536.2011.01924.x.
17. Bock M, Schmidt A, Bruckner T, et al. Occupational skin disease in the construction industry. Br J Dermatol 2003. https://doi.org/10.1111/j.1365-2133.2003.05748.x.
18. Aalto-Korte K, Alanko K, Kuuliala O, et al. Occupational methacrylate and acrylate allergy from glues. Contact Dermatitis 2008;58(6):340–6.
19. Liippo J, Lammintausta K. A case of occupational allergic contact dermatitis in a plumber performing pipeline repair. Contact Dermatitis 2011;65(4):247–8.
20. Reed J, Shaw S. Occupational allergic contact dermatitis in water-pipe renovators from diethylenetriamine in an epoxy resin system. Contact Dermatitis 1999. https://doi.org/10.1111/j.1600-0536.1999.tb06170.x.
21. Burnett CA, Lushniak BD, Mccarthy W, et al. Occupational dermatitis causing days away from work in U.S. private industry, 1993. Am J Ind Med 1998; 573:568–73.
22. Rietschel RL, Mathias CGT, Taylor JS, et al. A preliminary report of the occupation of patients evaluated in patch test clinics. Am J Contact Dermat 2001. https://doi.org/10.1053/ajcd.2001.19630.
23. Warshaw EM, Schram SE, Maibach HI, et al. Occupation-related contact dermatitis in North American health care workers referred for patch testing:

cross-sectional data, 1998 to 2004. Dermatitis 2008; 19(5):261–74.

24. Kadivar S, Belsito DV. Occupational dermatitis in health care workers evaluated for suspected allergic contact dermatitis. Dermatitis 2015;26(4):177–83.

25. Molin S, Bauer A, Schnuch A, et al. Occupational contact allergy in nurses: results from the Information Network of Departments of Dermatology 2003-2012. Contact Dermatitis 2015;72(3):164–71.

26. Suneja T, Belsito DV. Occupational dermatoses in health care workers evaluated for suspected allergic contact dermatitis. Contact Dermatitis 2008;58(5): 285–90.

27. Leggat PA, Kedjarune U, Smith DR. Occupational health problems in modern dentistry: a review. Ind Health 2007;45(5):611–21.

28. Lugović-Mihić L, Ferček I, Duvančić T, et al. Occupational contact dermatitis amongst dentists and dental technicians. Acta Clin Croat 2016;55(2): 293–300.

29. Wrangsjö K, Swartling C, Meding B. Occupational dermatitis in dental personnel: contact dermatitis with special reference to (meth)acrylates in 174 patients. Contact Dermatitis 2001;45(3):158–63.

30. Heratizadeh A, Werfel T, Schubert S, et al. Contact sensitization in dental technicians with occupational contact dermatitis. Data of the Information Network of Departments of Dermatology (IVDK) 2001–2015. Contact Dermatitis 2018;78(4):266–73.

31. Kocak O, Gul U. Patch test results of the dental personnel with contact dermatitis. Cutan Ocul Toxicol 2014;33(4):299–302.

32. Andreasson H, Boman A, Johnsson S, et al. On permeability of methyl methacrylate, 2-hydroxyethyl methacrylate and triethyleneglycol dimethacrylate through protective gloves in dentistry. Eur J Oral Sci 2003;111(6):529–35.

33. Thiboutot DM, Hamory BH, Marks JG. Dermatoses among floral shop workers. J Am Acad Dermatol 1990;22(1):54–8.

34. Santucci B, Picardo M, Iavarone C, et al. Contact dermatitis to Alstroemeria. Contact Dermatitis 1985. https://doi.org/10.1111/j.1600-0536.1985.tb01110.x.

35. Marks JG. Allergic contact dermatitis to alstroemeria. Arch Dermatol 1988. https://doi.org/10.1001/archderm.1988.01670060060017.

36. Bangha E, Elsner P. Occupational contact dermatitis toward sesquiterpene lactones in a florist. Am J Contact Dermat 1996. https://doi.org/10.1016/S1046-199X(96)90011-1.

37. Watanabe K, Yoshikawa K. Plant dermatitis seen in a florist. Ski Res 1983. https://doi.org/10.11340/skinresearch1959.25.660.

38. Schmidt RJ. Compositae. Clin Dermatol 1986. https://doi.org/10.1016/0738-081X(86)90063-5.

39. Tabar AI, Quirce S, García BE, et al. Primula dermatitis: versatility in its clinical presentation and the advantages of patch tests with synthetic primin. Contact Dermatitis 1994. https://doi.org/10.1111/j.1600-0536.1994.tb00734.x.

40. Hausen BM, Prater E, Schubert H. The sensitizing capacity of Alstroemeria cultivars in man and guinea pig: remarks on the occurrence, quantity and irritant and sensitizing potency of their constituents tuliposide A and tulipalin A (α-methylene-γ-butyrolactone). Contact Dermatitis 1983. https://doi.org/10.1111/j.1600-0536.1983.tb04625.x.

41. va der Walle HB, Brunsveld VM. Dermatitis in hairdressers: (I). The experience of the past 4 years. Contact Dermatitis 1994. https://doi.org/10.1111/j.1600-0536.1994.tb00647.x.

42. Hougaard MG, Winther L, Søsted H, et al. Occupational skin diseases in hairdressing apprentices - Has anything changed? Contact Dermatitis 2015; 72(1):40–6.

43. Warshaw EM, Wang MZ, Mathias T, et al. Occupational contact dermatitis in hairdressers/cosmetologists: retrospective analysis of North American contact dermatitis group data, 1994 to 2010. Dermatitis 2012;23(6):258–68.

44. Lyons G, Roberts H, Palmer A, et al. Hairdressers presenting to an occupational dermatology clinic in Melbourne, Australia. Contact Dermatitis 2013; 68(5):300–6.

45. Carøe TK, Ebbehøj NE, Agner T. Occupational dermatitis in hairdressers – influence of individual and environmental factors. Contact Dermatitis 2017;76(3):146–50.

46. Dahlquist I, Fregert S, Gruvberger B. Release of nickel from plated utensils in permanent wave liquids. Contact Dermatitis 1979. https://doi.org/10.1111/j.1600-0536.1979.tb05538.x.

47. Hansen KS. Occupational dermatoses in hospital cleaning women. Contact Dermatitis 1983;9(5): 343–51.

48. Singgih SIR, Lantinga H, Nater JP, et al. Occupational hand dermatoses in hospital cleaning personnel. Contact Dermatitis 1986;14(1):14–9.

49. Liskowsky J, Geier J, Bauer A. Contact allergy in the cleaning industry: analysis of contact allergy surveillance data of the Information Network of Departments of Dermatology. Contact Dermatitis 2011; 65(3):159–66.

50. Knudsen BB, Larsen E, Eusgaard H, et al. Release of thiurams and carbamates from rubber gloves. Contact Dermatitis 1993. https://doi.org/10.1111/j.1600-0536.1993.tb03343.x.

51. Meding B, Barregård L, Marcus K. Hand eczema in car mechanics. Contact Dermatitis 1994;30(3):129–34.

52. Warshaw EM, Hagen SL, Sasseville D, et al. Occupational contact dermatitis in mechanics and repairers referred for patch testing: retrospective analysis from the North American contact dermatitis group 1998-2014. Dermatitis 2017;28(1):47–57.

53. Attwa E, El-Laithy N. Contact dermatitis in car repair workers. J Eur Acad Dermatol Venereol 2009;23(2):138–45.

54. Suuronen K, Aalto-Korte K, Piipari R, et al. Occupational dermatitis and allergic respiratory diseases in Finnish metalworking machinists. Occup Med (Chic III) 2007;57(4):277–83.

55. Aalto-Korte K, Pesonen M, Suuronen K. Occupational allergic contact dermatitis caused by epoxy chemicals: occupations, sensitizing products, and diagnosis. Contact Dermatitis 2015. https://doi.org/10.1111/cod.12445.

56. Aalto-Korte K, Kuuliala O, Suuronen K, et al. Occupational contact allergy to formaldehyde and formaldehyde releasers. Contact Dermatitis 2008. https://doi.org/10.1111/j.1600-0536.2008.01422.x.

57. Warshaw EM, Hagen SL, DeKoven JG, et al. Occupational contact dermatitis in North American production workers referred for patch testing: retrospective analysis of cross-sectional data from the North American contact dermatitis group 1998 to 2014. Dermatitis 2017;28(3):183–94.

58. Warshaw EM, Hagen SL, Belsito DV, et al. Occupational contact dermatitis in North American print machine operators referred for patch testing: retrospective analysis of cross-sectional data from the North American contact dermatitis group 1998 to 2014. Dermatitis 2017;28(3):195–203.

59. Bauer A, Geier J, Elsner P, et al. Type IV allergy in the food processing industry: sensitization profiles in bakers, cooks and butchers. Contact Dermatitis 2002;46(4):228–35.

60. Warshaw EM, Kwon GP, Mathias CGT, et al. Occupationally related contact dermatitis in North American food service workers referred for patch testing, 1994 to 2010. Dermatitis 2013;24(1):22–8.

61. Gambichler T, Uzun A, Boms S, et al. Skin conditions in instrumental musicians: a self-reported survey. Contact Dermatitis 2008;58(4):217–22.

62. Kraft M, Schubert S, Geier J, et al. Contact dermatitis and sensitization in professional musicians. Contact Dermatitis 2019;80(5):273–8.

63. Lieberman HD, Fogelman JP, Ramsay DL, et al. Allergic contact dermatitis to propolis in a violin maker. J Am Acad Dermatol 2002;46(2 II):30–1.

64. Gamboa PM, Sánchez J, Segurola A, et al. Occupational contact dermatitis due to rosewood in a Basque wind instrument (txistu). Contact Dermatitis 2019;(July):1–2.

65. Lidén C, Kariberg A-T. Colophony in paper as a cause of hand eczema. Contact Dermatitis 1992;26(4):272–3.

The Importance of Education When Patch Testing

Peggy A. Wu, MD, MPH

KEYWORDS

- Patch test education • Patient education • Allergic contact dermatitis education
- Patch test training • Resources

KEY POINTS

- Before and while undergoing patch testing: Anticipate patients' patch test education needs before and during patch testing by presenting concise information about testing logistics and the concept of a delayed type hypersensitivity reaction. Review side effects with the expectation of experiencing common ones such as pruritus and tape irritation and putting rare but more serious adverse events in context.
- At the final patch testing reading: Set aside adequate time to verbally review a patient's relevant allergens, explaining their function, where they might be found, and potential cross reactors, and provide printed handouts to refer to later.
- A "safe list" of products that excludes a patient's relevant allergens and provides alternatives will increase their chances of successful avoidance.
- Be prepared to review and reinforce recommendations from the final patch reading at subsequent post patch testing visits, because patients' ability to accurately recall patch test results decreases with number of positives and time.

INTRODUCTION

Patient education is central to the implementation of a therapeutic plan that minimizes the chance of exposure to identified allergens and maximizes quality of life by allowing the patient agency in their daily lives. As such, the focus of this section is on the education of patients, who are presented a large volume of foreign information in a short period of time. This hurdle is made even more difficult because learning and implementing this information often occurs under challenging circumstances. Patients may have suffered for months to years dealing with anxiety, uncertainty, and helplessness regarding the cause of their distress. Their skin condition can have occupational consequences and contribute to stress around maintaining a livelihood. Sleep disturbance

is common, and personal and professional relationships are often impacted. Herein are presented strategies for optimizing education before, during, and after patch testing.

Understanding patterns of allergen exposure, potential cross-reactants, and strategies for allergen avoidance is a challenge for patients, contact dermatitis specialists, and allied health professionals alike. An additional update on patch testing resources and the state of contact dermatitis education in residency is provided.

PATIENT EDUCATION
Before Patch Testing

Patient education on patch testing can begin even before placement of the first patch test. Printed materials are often helpful to provide patients at

Department of Dermatology, University of California Davis, 3301 C Street, Suite 1400, Sacramento, CA 95816, USA
E-mail address: pawu@ucdavis.edu

Dermatol Clin 38 (2020) 351–360
https://doi.org/10.1016/j.det.2020.02.004
0733-8635/20/

the time of their consult visit or sent before their appointment with a description of patch testing, including logistical information such as the timing of appointments and restrictions of activity that would loosen the adherence of patches. This set of information helps the patient to optimize the logistical application of patches and their care to maximize the sensitivity and specificity at the time of reading.

A second set of information is required for expectation setting with regard to what is being tested and the potential side effects, as well as the likelihood of success in identifying relevant allergens. It may be helpful to emphasize during the consultation that the type of reaction that patch testing detects is a delayed reaction. Patients often associate patch testing that detects a delayed-type hypersensitivity reaction with prick, scratch, or intradermal testing that detects an immediate-type hypersensitivity reaction. It is important to clarify the differences and emphasize that patch testing is usually performed to identify the trigger of something that looks typically more like a scaly rash rather than shortness of breath, swelling, rhinorrhea, and so on. As such, it is acceptable to use antihistamines should patients feel itch or discomfort during the patch test process. Often it is important to clarify with patients that rather than dander or environmental or food protein allergies, patch testing identifies allergens that typically come in direct contact with the skin, with culprits such as fragrances, personal care products, metals, textiles, or rubber. It should also be emphasized for patients that, over the course of patch testing, they usually need to have 3 appointments for patches need to be placed, removed after 48 hours, and assessed at least twice (the preliminary and final patch test readings).

Expected side effects from patch testing include pruritus (which may be generalized), irritation from the tape, rash, and swelling at positive patch test reaction sites (**Table 1**). There are a few serious side effects associated with patch testing and those are infrequent. Occasionally, a positive reaction might be associated with a flare of the original skin reaction, particularly in patients who develop multiple positive reactions.[1] In some patients, confluent erythematous patches and plaques on the back can appear during patch testing, whereby it is impossible to distinguish between multiple true positive reactions and a generalized flare of rash. These results are both difficult to interpret and usually unreproducible. This is known as excited skin syndrome or angry back syndrome, and is more likely to occur in patients with active skin rashes that might involve the back.[2] Excited skin syndrome or angry back

Table 1	
Potential side effects of patch testing	
Common	**Rare**
Pruritus	Angry back syndrome
Tape irritation	Anaphylaxis
Rash at positive test sites	Infection
Postinflammatory changes at positive test sites	Scarring at site of positive patch reaction
Flare of rash with positive patch test	Sensitization

Adapted from Mowad CM, Anderson B, Scheinman P, et al. Allergic contact dermatitis: Patient management and education. J Am Acad Dermatol 2016;74(6):1048; with permission.

syndrome should not be confused with multiple positive reactions. The latter is more likely to appear as discrete lesions that are spaced apart and are reproducible. Separately, with individual reactions, the disrupted skin at a positive patch test site can infrequently become infected. In cases of infection, skin flora such as *Staphylococcus* or *Streptococcus* are the most likely causes, although one case of a deep fungal infection has been reported.[3]

Rarely, patients can develop a sensitization to patch test allergens and anaphylaxis has been reported. Sensitization to patch test reactions usually presents as a new, albeit delayed, reaction at the patch test site occurring 10 to 21 days after patch test application. This outcome can be confused with a persistent patch test reaction, which is a reaction that occurs during the first week of application but persists for 30 days or more. Gold is one of the most common culprits causing a persistent patch test reaction.[4] Other less likely causes can include phenylephrine, textile dyes, and methyl methacrylate.[5–7] Sensitization to allergens during patch testing is thought to be rare, but is likely underreported and is estimated to occur in approximately 0.1% of patch test patients. Paraphenylenediamine is one of the most common allergens reported to cause sensitization. Others include acrylates, epoxy resins, balsam of Peru, fragrance mix, composite mix, primula, and isothiazolinones.[4,8–14] Although it has been reported, anaphylaxis is exceedingly rare in patch testing and, if it were to occur, would typically do so within 30 minutes of application. The most common reported causative agent is ammonium persulfate, but formaldehyde, penicillin, bacitracin, disperse dye, and latex have also been described.[15–20]

By far the most common side effects of patch testing are pruritus, rash with positive patch test reactions, and irritant reaction to the tape. Following any skin inflammation, postinflammatory hyperpigmentation and hypopigmentation can occur, and, if there is enough disruption of the dermal epidermal junction, scarring. These common side effects of patch testing should be reviewed in detail during consultation before placement so that patients can understand what to expect. Uncommon side effects should also be mentioned and put in context. It is helpful to have a concise, printed handout that contains instructions as well as this information for patients to refer to later. In addition to printed materials, videos and photos can also be helpful in reviewing the patch test procedure.

The consultation visit is a good time to remind patients that patch testing does not always result in a positive, relevant reaction and subsequent diagnosis of allergic contact dermatitis (ACD). If no allergens are found, more testing may be needed. Based on the North American Contact Dermatitis Group data over the years, approximately two-thirds of patients will have at least one positive reaction, and the diagnosis of ACD is made in about 50% of patients who undergo patch testing.[21]

During Patch Testing

During patch, testing it is important to remind patients not to do any activities that might loosen contact between the patches and their skin. Activities such as bathing the patch test area, strenuous physical exercise, and swimming should be discouraged. Products are available to provide a waterproof covering or further secure patch tests if those activities cannot be avoided, but in general, to obtain the best results, patients should forgo any activities that would risk detachment of the patches.

Unless previously discussed, patients should be reminded that they should not start any new systemically or locally immunosuppressive therapies (oral steroids, methotrexate, cyclosporine, tacrolimus, mycophenolate mofetil, phototherapy, etc) while undergoing patch testing. **Table 2** shows a 2012 expert consensus of recommendations for managing immunomodulatory medications in patients undergoing patch testing.[22] However, patients can use oral antihistamines or cooling pads during testing to distract or decrease itch sensation.

Topical medicines, although okay to use on affected areas outside of the patch test area, should not be applied on sites undergoing patch testing 1 week before and during the patch test process. Phototherapy should also be withheld 1 week before patch testing and sunburn in the area of patch test application must also be avoided. However, using topical corticosteroids or steroid-sparing agents should be encouraged on any active rash sites outside of the patch test

Table 2
Approach to the patch test patient on immunomodulatory medications

Agent	Range of Recommendations	Consensus Opinion
Topical corticosteroids on test site	Avoid for 3–7 d	Evenly split between 3 and 7 d
UV exposure at test site	Avoid for 0 d to 2 wk	Avoid for 1 wk
Oral prednisone—maximum dosage	OK to test on 10–20 mg/d	OK to test on 10 mg, but best if able to DC
Oral prednisone withdrawal time	Avoid for 1–14 d	Avoid for 3–5 d
40 mg IM triamcinolone	Wait between 3 and 4 wk	Wait until 4 wk after injection
Methotrexate	Unknown to little/no effect	Little to no effect
TNF-α inhibitors	Unknown to little/no effect	Little to no effect
Ustekinumab	Unknown to little/no effect	Little to no effect
Azathioprine	Dose-dependent inhibition	Dose-dependent inhibition
Cyclosporine	Dose-dependent inhibition	Dose-dependent inhibition
Mycophenolate mofetil	Dose-dependent inhibition	Dose-dependent inhibition
Tacrolimus (systemic)	Dose-dependent inhibition	Dose-dependent inhibition

Results of poll of North American Contact Dermatitis Group members regarding effects of various agents on patch test reactions.
Abbreviations: d, day; DC, discontinue; IM, intramuscular; mg, milligram; TNF, tumor necrosis factor; UV, ultraviolet; wk, week.
From Fowler JF, Jr., Maibach HI, Zirwas M, et al. Effects of immunomodulatory agents on patch testing: expert opinion 2012. Dermatitis 2012;23(6):301; with permission.

area before and during patch testing, because there is evidence that active rash outside of patch test areas is associated with developing excited skin syndrome or angry back syndrome.[23]

Occasionally, patients are disappointed if at the preliminary patch test read, which usually occurs at the 48-hour removal of patches, there are no positive readings. Patients should be reminded that the final reading takes place more than 72 hours (usually 96 hours) from patch placement,[24] and ACD is a delayed reaction that may be negative at 48 hours but become positive at the final reading.

At the Final Patch Test Read

The final patch test reading is when the bulk of education about allergens identified during patch testing occurs. After an objective assessment is made of whether or not there is a reaction to the patch test, the most crucial part of the assessment takes place: determining of the relevance of each reaction. For each allergen deemed to be a positive reaction, relevance to the patient's current rash should be determined. Relevance can be labeled as past or current. Current relevance is further delineated as possible (when the patient is exposed to skin contact with the type of materials that may contain the allergen), probable (if the allergen is identified as an ingredient or component of a contactant used by the patient), or of definite relevance. Definite relevance typically requires testing to the actual product, removing it with improvement, and reintroducing the rash with exposure. Items can be of past relevance if the person is no longer using the contactant with the allergen but has a history of use and subsequent development of a rash.

Sometimes, if the relevance of an allergen is not clear, patients can try a use test such as the repeated open application test, whereby the patient uses the product containing the allergen as is (if it is a leave-on product, it is left on; if it is wash or cleanser, washed off or diluted 1:10) twice a day on an unaffected area of skin for 2 to 4 weeks.[25]

Another way to determine the relevance of a patch test reaction is by reviewing the patient's products. This review can be done by having the patient take photos of the ingredients of the personal care products that they use, transcribing the ingredient lists of their products, or by bringing in the products themselves to examine for ingredients. This process also helps to instruct patients on how to read labels and look for their identified allergens.

To aid patients in understanding their reactions and recall allergens, it is helpful to group allergens by functional categories (**Fig. 1**).[4] For example, fragrance, balsam of Peru, as well as ylang ylang oil, lavender, cinnamic aldehyde can be grouped into substances that impart a pleasant odor to personal care products. Similarly, tixocortol pivalate, clobetasol, and budesonide are cortisone allergens; and thiuram mix, carba mix, black rubber mix, and mercaptobenzothiazole are rubber accelerators.

However, sometimes allergens have more than one function and can be found in multiple places. For example, formaldehyde can be used in textiles, including 100% cotton, to prevent wrinkling, and it is also a preservative used in personal care products. Another potential pitfall is that even items labeled as fragrance free or for sensitive skin are often not actually fragrance free. It is legal to use the term fragrance free in a product that contains fragrance if those ingredients are not used solely to impart an odor to a product, but have other functions such as emollients or preservatives.[26] One example of this is benzyl alcohol, which is a fragrance and a preservative.

At the final patch test reading, patients should understand the use and nature of their relevant allergens, where they can be found, and potential cross-reactors. Often, this process requires a thorough discussion and printed materials to review. Providers must allocate enough time for this discussion because the key to successful avoidance and prevention of ACD is patient education.

Resources

There are several resources available to help patients and practitioners navigate a patients' relevant patch test results. Handouts in both English and Spanish are available from the American Contact Dermatitis Society (ACDS) website (www.contactderm.org); textbooks, such as *Contact and Occupational Dermatology*, have patient handouts with information on common allergens. Manufactures of patch test materials such as Chemotechnique (www.chemotechnique.se); Smartpractice, which makes other the preloaded, US Food and Drug Administration-approved T.R.U.E. TEST, as well as expanded patch series (www.truetest.com; www.smartpractice.com) have printable materials on allergens. Websites like the Dermatitis Academy (www.dermatitis academy.com) also have videos available to describe specific allergens and the patch test process.

When providing patients information about their patch testing results, cognitive theory would recommend minimizing extraneous information.[4] One or 2 sentences describing each allergen

Category	Patch test allergen
Fragrances	Fragrance mix
	M. pereirae resin (balsam of Peru)
	Fragrance mix II
	Cinnamal (cinnamic aldehyde)
Preservatives	Methylisothiazolinone
	Formaldehyde
	Methylchloroisothiazolinone/methylisothiazolinone
	Iodopropynyl butylcarbamate
	Quaternium-15
	Methyldibromoglutaronitrile/phenoxyethanol
Surfactants	Oleamidopropyl dimethylamine
	Dimethylaminopropylamine
	Decyl glucoside
	Cocamidopropyl betaine
Botanicals	Propolis
	Compositae mix
Hair	4-Phenylenediamine base
	Ammonium persulfate
Sun protection	Benzophenone-4
	Propylene glycol
	Lanolin alcohol
Metal	Nickel
	Cobalt
	Potassium dichromate
Rubber accelerator	Carba mix
	Thiuram mix
	Diphenylguanidine
Adhesive	2-HEMA
	Colophonium
	Bisphenol A epoxy resin
	Ethyl acrylate
Medicaments	Neomycin
	Bacitracin
	Tixocortol-21-pivalate
	Benzocaine
	Most often found in personal care products
	Metal
	Rubber accelerator – could be occupational
	Adhesive
	Medicament (includes antibiotics and steroids)

Fig. 1. North American contact dermatitis group top 35 common allergens grouped by category. (*From* DeKoven JG, Warshaw EM, Zug KA, et al. North American Contact Dermatitis Group Patch Test Results: 2015-2016. Dermatitis 2018;29(6):297-309; with permission.)

verbally, combined with a concise printed handout, seems to be most effective. The risk of information overload be kept in mind when explaining particular allergens and potential cross-reactions, because the volume of material presented at the final patch test reading can be daunting. Printed health care materials for patients should be understandable at a 6th grade or lower reading level. It can be helpful to provide patients concrete tools to put clinical recommendations into practice and thereby increase actionability.[4] One way to do this is to demonstrate how to read labels to avoid culprit allergens and make sure that patients have a follow-up plan in place. However, patients should be aware that allergens can have multiple names as well as potential cross-reactors, such as formaldehyde and formaldehyde-releasing preservatives, which cross-react 36% of the time.[27]

Because of the potential pitfalls of reading labels, it is important to be able to provide patients safe alternatives to the products they can no longer use. There are 2 large databases that can provide such lists. These are the Contact Allergen Management Program and SkinSAFE. The Contact Allergen Management Program is a member benefit of the ACDS and contains more than 7000 products that are updated every 6 months to a year. SkinSAFE is a for-profit site available via subscription by month or year for health care professionals and patients. By entering a list of allergens to which a patient is allergic, these websites generate lists of safe products in every category to choose as alternatives. One tip to increase actionability is to help the patient choose 1 item from each category they will need to replace. There is evidence that using a safe list increases the odds of successful avoidance of culprit allergens.[28–30] Another potential benefit is that it has been shown to save counseling time at the final patch test reading.[31] Ideally, patients are presented both information explaining culprit allergens, how to identify those allergens in their personal care products or daily lives, as well as a safe list of alternatives at their final patch test reading.

Finally, it is important for the patch test practitioner to help the patient put their patch test reactions and diagnosis of ACD in context with any other existing skin issues. It is not uncommon for there to be concomitant dermatologic diagnoses within the same patient, such as atopic dermatitis and ACD, or irritant contact dermatitis with ACD, or even lichen planus or psoriasis with ACD. Dermatologists and other skin care providers are uniquely able to help patients distinguish between potentially overlapping presentations of competing diagnoses. The identity of the relevant allergens and subsequent discussion with the patient and materials provided should all be documented in the medical record and shared with the patient's primary dermatologist and/or primary care provider to facilitate communication and care.

After Patch Testing

After patch testing, it can be helpful to have patients follow up anywhere between 2-4 months from their final patch test reading with the patch test provider or their primary dermatologist to ensure that any questions regarding patch testing results or lingering dermatitis issues do not remain. Contact with culprit allergens should generally be

avoided for 2 months to ensure an adequate wash out period before reassessment. At the follow-up visit, providers should be prepared to review much of the information that was given at the final patch test reading, including a patient's allergens and where those allergens can be found. Several studies have demonstrated that a patient's ability to retain information, especially about multiple positive and relevant reactions, deteriorates over time[30,32] (**Fig. 2**).

Throughout the patch test process, practitioners can engage patient involvement as well as assess their level of understanding by asking patients questions about their familiarity with contact dermatitis and goals of patch testing, as well as assessing impact on quality of life. **Table 3** shows example questions of how to prompt discussion and assess education levels regarding ACD before and after patch testing.[33]

If patients are not improved with avoidance of their identified allergens, one should consider other potential sources of a culprit allergen, or additional workup. Another possible source of exposure might be a person's close contacts, so-called connubial or consort ACD. This possibility should be especially considered when the patient is a caretaker for another person or pet. Systemic contact dermatitis could also be considered especially if the patient has a reaction to nickel or balsam of Peru, two of the most common causes of systemic contact dermatitis.[34] If the rash is in a symmetric presentation, generalized, or has a pomphylox or dyshidrotic eczema appearance, in the case of a positive patch test to nickel, one should consider recommending a low nickel diet. There is a published point system guide to help patients to adhere to a low nickel diet.[35] If patients have perioral or perianal disease and a positive

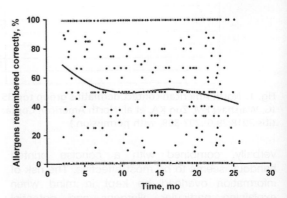

Fig. 2. Percentage of allergens recalled correctly over time. (*From* Scalf LA, Genebriera J, Davis MDP, et al. Patients' perceptions of the usefulness and outcome of patch testing. J Am Acad Dermatol 2007;56(6):931; with permission.)

Table 3
Questions to ask patients to prompt discussion

Timing of Questions	Suggested Questions to Prompt Discussion
At patch test consultation	What do you think is causing your rash? How familiar are you with contact dermatitis/patch testing?
At the final reading, after avoidance education	What will you remember from this visit? How confident are you that you can avoid your allergens?
At follow-up visit	What allergens do you avoid? What advice would you give to a patient who is in a similar situation?

Data from DeKoven JG, Warshaw EM, Zug KA, et al. North American Contact Dermatitis Group Patch Test Results: 2015-2016. Dermatitis 2018;29(6):297-309.

reaction to balsam of Peru, a low balsam of Peru diet should be considered. In one series, 47% of fragrance allergic patients improved on a low Balsam of Peru diet.[36] Because dietary changes can be onerous, it is usually recommended to start with 1 month. Other potential diagnoses include photoallergic contact dermatitis, particularly if the patient has a distribution on the face, neck, upper extremities, and upper chest; this diagnosis could be verified with photopatch testing.

Depending on the number of allergens placed, it is possible that additional allergy tests should be done. Some studies have shown that the T.R.U.E. test alone can miss up to 50% of relevant allergens, and even the extended series without additional trays could leave out relevant reactions.[37,38] If the rash suspected of being ACD persists despite comprehensive patch testing that does not adequately explain the rash, further workup should be considered, including blood tests (ie, complete blood count, comprehensive metabolic panel) or skin biopsy.[39]

On a population level, primary, secondary, and tertiary prevention measures have been examined for contact dermatitis predominantly in the occupational setting. Primary prevention is aimed at averting healthy individuals from developing contact dermatitis; secondary prevention is meant to improve early diagnosis and intervention. Tertiary prevention addresses individuals with more advanced presentations of contact dermatitis. Guiding principles of primary prevention starting as early in training as possible are increasing knowledge about skin diseases; education emphasizing skin protection such as reducing handwashing and increasing moisturization; and encouraging the use of protective measures like gloves. Internationally, several primary prevention programs have been implemented for different occupations including hairdressers, health care workers, and bakers with varying success.[40] Secondary and tertiary prevention programs have also been implemented in programs and seminars aimed at particular occupations or presentations, such as hand dermatitis.[41]

EDUCATION OF PROVIDERS
When to Refer to Patch Testing

It is important to educate skin care practitioners on how to recognize when patch testing may be necessary and how to best manage patients who have had patch testing. Patch testing should be considered when a patient with a previously well-controlled rash experiences an ongoing flare, such as a patient with atopic dermatitis who suddenly worsens and continues to have uncontrolled disease despite adequate treatment for the flare, or if the dermatitis manifests in an atypical atopic dermatitis distribution or in a pattern suggestive of contact dermatitis such as eyelid predominance, perioral predominance, genital predominance head and neck predominance, hand and foot predominance.[42] In addition to patients with chronic dermatitis, other potential ACD cases are patients who have never experienced a rash and develop an ongoing, perhaps waxing and waning rash that may respond to treatment but returns once treatment is discontinued. Another scenario one might consider patch testing is before starting an immunosuppressive or immunomodulating agent if ACD is on the differential diagnosis. Medications such as prednisone at doses of more than 10 mg, mycophenolate mofetil, cyclosporine, and azathioprine have been known to suppress positive responses to patch testing. Even dupilumab, the IL-4 and IL-13 inhibitor targeting the T helper 2 axis, has been reported to alter the patch test response to nickel in nickel-allergic patients.[43]

Training Future Patch Test Practitioners

Even if the skin care provider does not perform patch testing themselves, by familiarizing themselves with the process they will be able to identify patients who would benefit from patch testing as well as support them through the process of identifying and avoiding culprit allergens. Patients overwhelmingly benefit from patch testing, with more than 81% reporting improvement after patch testing and multiple studies demonstrating cost effectiveness and improvement in quality of life.[44,45] However, patch testing is time consuming and requires additional training.

Across specialties of dermatology and allergy, survey studies have shown that a major determinant of whether someone will pursue a career that encompasses patch testing is a function of their exposure during training.[46–48] A 2010 survey of US dermatology residencies revealed that approximately 82% to 85% of programs report patch testing available as a diagnostic tool in use in their clinics and only 22% to 27% report a dedicated patch testing rotation.[49] These numbers have not significantly changed since the initial survey 7 years prior.[50] Sixty-one percent of program directors and chief residents of dermatology programs recalled having a patch testing expert within their faculty, most of whom are affiliated with ACDS. There is a need to increase exposure to patch testing techniques to train the future generation of patch testers. The ACDS holds an annual meeting before the American Academy of Dermatology with yearly alternating basic and advanced education tracks for patch test providers as well as a meeting in the fall. Dermatologists are uniquely equipped to ensure the appropriate use, execution, interpretation of patch testing, and subsequent education to diagnose and successfully manage ACD. Furthermore, dermatologists' training and skills allow them to distinguish between, identify overlap, and tease out relationships between concomitant skin disorders.

SUMMARY

The cornerstone of managing ACD is avoidance of allergens, and a key part of avoidance is understanding one's patch test results and the implications. It is important for patients to understand these reactions because 88% of reactions found on patch testing will be retained over time.[51] Whereas the majority of patients report improvement after patch testing, other studies have shown that there is room for progress in areas, such as patient recall of allergens.[30,43,52] This article has outlined several resources, techniques, and tips to use before, during and after patch testing to aid the practitioner in educating patch test patients about their ACD and maximize their opportunity for successful management.

ACKNOWLEDGMENTS

The author thanks Dr Victor Huang for his insightful edits and comments.

DISCLOSURE

The author has nothing to disclose.

REFERENCES

1. Mose AP, Steenfeldt N, Andersen KE. Flare-up of dermatitis following patch testing is more common in polysensitized patients. Contact Dermatitis 2010; 63(5):289–90.
2. Mitchell J, Maibach HI. Managing the excited skin syndrome: patch testing hyperirritable skin. Contact Dermatitis 1997;37(5):193–9.
3. Lesueur BW, Warschaw K, Fredrikson L. Necrotizing cellulitis caused by Apophysomyces elegans at a patch test site. Am J Contact Dermat 2002;13(3): 140–2.
4. Mowad CM, Anderson B, Scheinman P, et al. Allergic contact dermatitis: patient management and education. J Am Acad Dermatol 2016;74(6): 1043–54.
5. Patrizi A, Lanzarini M, Tosti A. Persistent patch test reactions to textile dyes. Contact Dermatitis 1990; 23(1):60–1.
6. Corazza M, Virgili A, Martina S. Allergic contact stomatitis from methyl methacrylate in a dental prosthesis, with a persistent patch test reaction. Contact Dermatitis 1992;26(3):210–1.
7. Rafael M, Pereira F, Faria MA. Allergic contact blepharoconjunctivitis caused by phenylephrine, associated with persistent patch test reaction. Contact Dermatitis 1998;39(3):143–4.
8. Hillen U, Dickel H, Loffler H, et al. Late reactions to patch test preparations with reduced concentrations of p-phenylenediamine: a multicentre investigation of the German Contact Dermatitis Research Group. Contact Dermatitis 2011;64(4):196–202.
9. Hillen U, Frosch PJ, Franckson T, et al. Optimizing the patch-test concentration of para-tertiary-butylcatechol: results of a prospective study with a dilution series. Contact Dermatitis 2003;48(3):140–3.
10. Hillen U, Frosch PJ, John SM, et al. Patch test sensitization caused by para-tertiary-butylcatechol. Results of a prospective study with a dilution series. Contact Dermatitis 2001;45(4):193–6.
11. Hillen U, Jappe U, Frosch PJ, et al. Late reactions to the patch-test preparations para-phenylenediamine and epoxy resin: a prospective multicentre investigation of the German Contact Dermatitis Research Group. Br J Dermatol 2006;154(4):665–70.
12. Kanerva L, Estlander T, Alanko K, et al. Patch test sensitization to Compositae mix, sesquiterpene-lactone mix, Compositae extracts, laurel leaf,

Chlorophorin, Mansonone A, and dimethoxydalbergione. Am J Contact Dermat 2001;12(1):18–24.

13. Isaksson M, Gruvberger B. Patch test sensitization to methylchloroisothiazolinone + methylisothiazolinone and 4,4'-diaminodiphenylmethane. Contact Dermatitis 2003;48(1):53–4.

14. Wilkinson SM, Pollock B. Patch test sensitization after use of the Compositae mix. Contact Dermatitis 1999;40(5):277–8.

15. Haustein UF. Anaphylactic shock and contact urticaria after the patch test with professional allergens. Allerg Immunol (Leipz) 1976;22(4):349–52.

16. Hoekstra M, van der Heide S, Coenraads PJ, et al. Anaphylaxis and severe systemic reactions caused by skin contact with persulfates in hair-bleaching products. Contact Dermatitis 2012;66(6):317–22.

17. Orlandini A, Viotti G, Magno L. Anaphylactoid reaction induced by patch testing with formaldehyde in an asthmatic. Contact Dermatitis 1988;19(5):383–4.

18. Parry EJ, Beck MH. Acute anaphylaxis resulting from routine patch testing with latex. Contact Dermatitis 1999;41(4):236–7.

19. Perfetti L, Galdi E, Biale C, et al. Anaphylactoid reaction to patch testing with ammonium persulfate. Allergy 2000;55(1):94–5.

20. Washio K, Ijuin K, Fukunaga A, et al. Contact anaphylaxis caused by Basic Blue 99 in hair dye. Contact Dermatitis 2017;77(2):122–3.

21. DeKoven JG, Warshaw EM, Zug KA, et al. North American contact dermatitis group patch test results: 2015-2016. Dermatitis 2018;29(6):297–309.

22. Fowler JF Jr, Maibach HI, Zirwas M, et al. Effects of immunomodulatory agents on patch testing: expert opinion 2012. Dermatitis 2012;23(6):301–3.

23. Magembe AJ, Davis MD, Richardson DM. A localized flare of dermatitis may render patch tests uninterpretable in some patients with recently controlled widespread dermatitis. Dermatitis 2009;20(5):261–4.

24. Johansen JD, Aalto-Korte K, Agner T, et al. European Society of Contact Dermatitis guideline for diagnostic patch testing - recommendations on best practice. Contact Dermatitis 2015;73(4):195–221.

25. Brown GE, Botto N, Butler DC, et al. Clinical utilization of repeated open application test among American Contact Dermatitis Society Members. Dermatitis 2015;26(5):224–9.

26. Katta R. Common misconceptions in contact dermatitis counseling. Dermatol Online J 2008;14(4):2.

27. Fasth IM, Ulrich NH, Johansen JD. Ten-year trends in contact allergy to formaldehyde and formaldehyde-releasers. Contact Dermatitis 2018;79(5):263–9.

28. Edman B. The usefulness of detailed information to patients with contact allergy. Contact Dermatitis 1988;19(1):43–7.

29. Caperton C, Jacob SE. Improving post-patch-test education with the contact allergen replacement database. Dermatitis 2007;18(2):101–2.

30. Scalf LA, Genebriera J, Davis MD, et al. Patients' perceptions of the usefulness and outcome of patch testing. J Am Acad Dermatol 2007;56(6):928–32.

31. Kist JM, el-Azhary RA, Hentz JG, et al. The contact allergen replacement database and treatment of allergic contact dermatitis. Arch Dermatol 2004;140(12):1448–50.

32. Jamil WN, Lindberg M. Effects of time and recall of patch test results on quality of life (QoL) after testing. Cross-sectional study analyzing QoL in hand eczema patients 1, 5 and 10 years after patch testing. Contact Dermatitis 2017;77(2):88–94.

33. Smith MC. Patient education to enhance contact dermatitis evaluation and testing. Dermatol Clin 2009;27(3):323–7, vii.

34. Fabbro SK, Zirwas MJ. Systemic contact dermatitis to foods: nickel, BOP, and more. Curr Allergy Asthma Rep 2014;14(10):463.

35. Mislankar M, Zirwas MJ. Low-nickel diet scoring system for systemic nickel allergy. Dermatitis 2013;24(4):190–5.

36. Salam TN, Fowler JF Jr. Balsam-related systemic contact dermatitis. J Am Acad Dermatol 2001;45(3):377–81.

37. Patel D, Belsito DV. The detection of clinically relevant contact allergens with a standard screening tray of 28 allergens. Contact Dermatitis 2012;66(3):154–8.

38. Larkin A, Rietschel RL. The utility of patch tests using larger screening series of allergens. Am J Contact Dermat 1998;9(3):142–5.

39. Spiker A, Mowad CM. Evaluation and Management of Patch Test-Negative Patients With Generalized Dermatitis. Dermatitis 2017;28(4):261–4. https://doi.org/10.1097/DER.0000000000000282.

40. Bauer A, Ronsch H, Elsner P, et al. Interventions for preventing occupational irritant hand dermatitis. Cochrane Database Syst Rev 2018;(4):CD004414.

41. Seyfarth F, Schliemann S, Antonov D, et al. Teaching interventions in contact dermatitis. Dermatitis 2011;22(1):8–15.

42. Chen JK, Jacob SE, Nedorost ST, et al. A Pragmatic Approach to Patch Testing Atopic Dermatitis Patients: Clinical Recommendations Based on Expert Consensus Opinion. Dermatitis 2016;27(4):186–92.

43. Zhu GA, Chen JK, Chiou A, et al. Repeat patch testing in a patient with allergic contact dermatitis improved on dupilumab. JAAD Case Rep 2019;5(4):336–8.

44. Steuer MS, Botto NC. Patient reported improvement after patch testing and allergen avoidance counseling: a retrospective analysis. Dermatol Ther (Heidelb) 2018;8(3):435–40.

45. Ramirez F, Chren MM, Botto N. A review of the impact of patch testing on quality of life in allergic contact dermatitis. J Am Acad Dermatol 2017; 76(5):1000–4.

46. James WD, Rosenthal LE, Brancaccio RR, et al. American Academy of Dermatology Patch Testing Survey: use and effectiveness of this procedure. J Am Acad Dermatol 1992;26(6):991–4.

47. Ghaffari G, Craig T. The perceived obstacles in performing patch test to detect allergic contact dermatitis: a comparison between community allergists and directors of allergy training programs. Ann Allergy Asthma Immunol 2008;100(4):323–6.

48. Fonacier L, Charlesworth EM, Mak WY, et al. American College of Allergy, Asthma & Immunology Patch Testing and Allergic Dermatologic Disease Survey: use of patch testing and effect of education on

49. Nelson J, Mowad C, Sun H. Allergic contact dermatitis and patch-testing education in US dermatology residencies in 2010. Dermatitis 2012;23(2):56–60.

50. High WA, Cruz PD Jr. Contact dermatitis education in dermatology residency programs: can (will) the American Contact Dermatitis Society be a force for improvement? Am J Contact Dermat 2003;14(4): 195–9.

51. Ayala F, Balato N, Lembo G, et al. Statistical evaluation of the persistence of acquired hypersensitivity by standardized patch tests. Contact Dermatitis 1996;34(5):354–8.

52. Lewis FM, Cork MJ, McDonagh AJ, et al. An audit of the value of patch testing: the patient's perspective. Contact Dermatitis 1994;30(4):214–6.

confidence, attitude, and usage. Am J Contact Dermat 2002;13(4):164–9.

Orthopedic Implant Hypersensitivity Reactions
Concepts and Controversies

Matthew Barrett Innes, MD[a], Amber Reck Atwater, MD[b],*

KEYWORDS

- Implant hypersensitivity reaction • Orthopedic implant • Metal hypersensitivity reaction
- Allergic contact dermatitis • Type IV hypersensitivity reaction • Metal allergy • Implant allergy

KEY POINTS

- Clinical presentations of implant hypersensitivity reactions (IHRs) include localized and generalized cutaneous reactions and noncutaneous complications. Localized dermatitis directly overlying the implanted material is the most supportive of IHRs.
- Orthopedic implants usually include metals and also may contain nonmetal components, such as bone cement, plastics, and ceramics.
- The pathogenesis of IHRs is still being investigated but likely includes both a type IV delayed hypersensitivity reaction as well as the innate immune response.
- The best diagnostic test for IHRs is patch testing, and routine preimplant patch testing is not recommended. Postimplant patch testing can be completed when symptoms are consistent with a potential IHRs.
- Diagnostic criteria can help with determination as to whether orthopedic implant symptoms are due to IHRs.

INTRODUCTION

There is a growing concern over hypersensitivity reactions to implanted devices. This is, in part, because of the aging population and associated increasing number of implanted devices. As awareness of the potential for allergic reactions to these implanted devices has increased, so have referrals to dermatologists for preimplantation and postimplantation patch testing as well as questions from patients regarding their potential risk of allergy-related complications. Although not all dermatologists perform patch testing, this is an issue likely to come up in every dermatology practice. For example, patients might ask if their history of reacting to jewelry indicates a need for preimplant patch testing or if their nickel allergy could be causing their implant complications.

Numerous cases of hypersensitivity reactions to implanted devices have been reported and this topic is complex and controversial. Metals are implicated most commonly, but other allergens also have been reported. Implant hypersensitivity reactions (IHRs) also have been reported with orthopedic, dental, cardiovascular, and gynecologic implants as well as with various clips, plates, and other hardware and devices. This review focuses on orthopedic IHRs and their associated concepts and controversies.

CLINICAL PRESENTATION OF IMPLANT HYPERSENSITIVITY REACTIONS

Clinically relevant orthopedic IHRs are rare but do occur. It is common enough for providers and patients to question whether cutaneous

[a] Tanner Clinic, 2121 North 1700 West, Layton, UT 84041, USA; [b] Duke Dermatology, 5324 McFarland Road #210, Durham, NC 27707, USA
* Corresponding author.
E-mail address: amber.atwater@duke.edu

Dermatol Clin 38 (2020) 361–369
https://doi.org/10.1016/j.det.2020.02.005
0733-8635/20/© 2020 Elsevier Inc. All rights reserved.

and even noncutaneous concerns could be related to recently implanted devices. It, therefore, is vital for dermatologists to have an understanding of potential clinical presentations of IHRs so that informed discussion and counseling can occur. The 3 main reaction patterns in reported cases of implant-related hypersensitivity reactions are localized dermatitis, generalized dermatitis, and extracutaneous complications.

Localized Cutaneous Implant Hypersensitivity Reactions

Localized cutaneous reactions receive the most scientific support in the literature. These typically are eczematous in nature and overlie the implanted material. For example, Thomas and colleagues[1] reported a case of right lower leg dermatitis after plate fixation for tibial fracture. Patch testing confirmed nickel allergy, and the plate was removed. The dermatitis persisted, however, and this was attributed to a broken drill bit that had been purposefully left in place to avoid tibial trauma. Gao and colleagues[2] described a patient who underwent total knee arthroplasty (TKA) with a cobalt-chromium-molybdenum prosthesis and subsequently developed eczema around the operative scar, followed by generalized eczema. Postoperative patch testing revealed a positive patch test reaction to chromium. He underwent revision surgery, with resolution of his pruritus within 3 days and of his eczema within 2 months. Similarly, Treudler and Simon[3] reported a case of right leg dermatitis overlying an implant; benzoyl peroxide (from bone cement) was implicated.

Generalized Cutaneous Implant Hypersensitivity Reactions

Generalized eruptions are less common in the literature. One case from 1972 describes a patient with diffuse eczematous dermatitis attributed to stainless steel orthopedic screws.[4] The surgeon "begrudgingly" removed the screws, and within 72 hours the dermatitis and pruritus resolved. The patient had positive patch test reactions to nickel and pieces of the screw, which contained 14% nickel. Another case documents diffuse nummular dermatitis that occurred 3 weeks after implantation of a titanium-vanadium-aluminum alloy plate in the foot; patch testing was positive for vanadium, and the dermatitis cleared within 3 weeks of plate removal.[5] Other reported cutaneous reactions include urticarial, bullous, and vasculitic eruptions.[6]

Extracutaneous Complications of Orthopedic Implants

Extracutaneous complications that have been associated with IHRs include implant loosening and failure, implant-site pain and swelling, delayed healing, aseptic lymphocytic vasculitis-associated lesions, and local pseudotumor growth.[7] These complications, and whether they are due to delayed-type hypersensitivity reactions, tend to be more controversial in the literature.

PATHOGENESIS OF IMPLANT HYPERSENSITIVITY REACTIONS

Implanted orthopedic devices are exposed to biological fluids and tissues and to mechanical strain, and as a result they experience degradation, corrosion, and wear. These can result in the release of metal ions and wear particles. The release of metal ions, and their subsequent exposure to the local immune system, are important concepts in the discussion of the pathogenesis of implant-related hypersensitivity reactions.

The traditional paradigm for the pathogenesis of allergic contact dermatitis is a type IV delayed hypersensitivity reaction, which involves a cutaneous sensitization phase followed by an elicitation phase. It is unclear as to what degree the allergic pathways in the peri-implant tissues mirror this traditional immunologic pathway. When the suspected allergen is a metal in an implant, the sensitization phase occurs in a different microenvironment, with a complement of immune cells different from those found in the skin. Thus, it is likely that the pathogenesis of metal implant hypersensitivity does not completely parallel the traditional pathway of allergic contact dermatitis. It is known that noncutaneous exposure can lead to elicitation of systemic contact dermatitis, such as when ingested allergens cause diffuse cutaneous and sometimes extracutaneous findings. It is possible that peri-implant tissues could act as the site of sensitization, particularly with the corrosion and wear that take place with implanted devices. It also is possible, however, that very different immunologic responses take place in this peri-implant environment.

Schalock and colleagues[8] suggest that the peri-implant immunologic reaction is multifactorial and includes both innate and acquired immune system activation. This concept is supported in a recent study by Christiansen and colleagues.[9] Their group compared peri-implant tissue metal concentrations and cytokine profiles for 3 total hip replacement groups:

1. Revision for aseptic loosening, osteolysis, or unexplainable pain
2. Revision for fracture, dislocation, or component failure
3. Primary total hip replacement (control)

Metal concentrations were increased in peri-implant tissue for both revision groups, and the aseptic loosening group exhibited a cytokine profile with increased levels of interleukin (IL)-1, IL-8, and tumor necrosis factor α, consistent with an innate immune response and increased levels of IL-2 and interferon γ, which is more consistent with a T-cell–mediated response.

Numerous reports document the presence of elevated metal ion levels in the serum of patients with failing metal implants.[10–17] Some studies also report elevated levels in urine, synovial fluid, lymph nodes, and internal organs.[18,19] For example, Savarino and colleagues[17] described 59 patients with TKA, 24 with stable implants and 35 with failing implants. Serum ion levels of aluminum, titanium, chromium, and cobalt were measured in both groups as well as in 41 controls. Chromium levels were significantly elevated in patients with failing implants ($P = .001$), with mean serum levels approximately twice as high as in the stable implant and control groups. Some investigators suspect that these higher serum and tissue levels of metals are associated with an increased risk of hypersensitivity reactions. Others believe that elevated metal levels could be the result of joint failure rather than the cause or that the elevated levels do mark joint failure but do not herald the development of hypersensitivity. Likewise, some suggest that a peri-implant lymphocytic infiltrate may represent an immunologic response without necessarily equating to a delayed-type hypersensitive reaction.[20]

Implants can fail for a variety of reasons, including aseptic osteolysis, infection, recurrent dislocation, fracture, and surgical error.[10,21–23] This, in combination with the fact that positive patch test reactions are relatively common in the general population, can make it difficult to rule in or rule out a true causal association. It is clear that more research on the pathogenesis of IHRs is needed.

ORTHOPEDIC IMPLANT COMPONENTS

In the context of IHRs, investigators typically include both dynamic and static orthopedic implanted devices. Dynamic implants are moveable, for example, knees and hips. In the 1960s,

metal-on-metal dynamic implants were introduced; these had high rates of metal ion release and sensitization.[6] Metal-on-plastic implants also are available and reportedly have a lower risk of metal ion release. Second-generation metal-on-metal implants are now available, and there have been some reports of metals present in the urine and serum of these patients.[13,15] Static implanted materials typically are predominantly metal and include materials like plates and screws.

Metals

The bulk of the literature discussing orthopedic IHRs focuses on metal allergens. Allergic contact dermatitis to metals generally occurs only when metal salts are in solution. In the skin, this occurs when metals come in contact with sweat or other body fluids.[24] Metal implants are subject to an unusually intense and prolonged exposure to body fluids, increasing the risk of corrosion of the metal and subsequent exposure to metal salts, theoretically increasing the risk of sensitization.

Total knee implants comprise 3 components: femur, tibia, and patella. Total hip implants comprise a femoral stem, femoral head, and acetabular cup. The most common metals used in modern hip and knee implants are cobalt-chromium alloys, titanium, and titanium alloys. Metals, such as vanadium and molybdenum, can be added to these alloys to boost their strength or improve corrosion resistance.[25] Oxidized zirconium has been used more recently as a hypoallergenic option in patients allergic to nickel.[8]

In knee and hip implants, titanium is utilized in the form of commercially pure titanium or an alloy of titanium-aluminum-vanadium. Titanium has the best record for osseointegration, which refers to the integration of surrounding bone into the implant.[26] IHRs to titanium is exceedingly rare, but reports of suspected IHRs to titanium are present in the literature. Wood and Warshaw[27] provided a thorough review of hypersensitivity reactions to titanium and summarized reported cases of titanium IHRs in orthopedic and other implanted devices. Some investigators recommend using titanium implants on a preventive basis for patients at risk for IHRs. The German Implant Allergy Working Group proposed that titanium-based osteosynthesis materials be used for all metal-allergic patients, negating the need for preimplant allergy testing.[28] The American Contact Dermatitis Society (ACDS) also recommends the use of titanium when preimplant testing is not performed in a patient with self-reported metal allergy or when preimplant testing is recommended but is not possible or is refused.[8]

Stainless steel is an iron-based alloy that is commonly used in static implants and hardware, such as plates and screws for internal fixation of fractures; Society of Automotive Engineers (SAE) 316L is referred to as *surgical steel* and is the most common variety used in medical applications due to its high chromium content, which imparts corrosion resistance. Other ingredients include nickel, cobalt, molybdenum, and other trace metals.[6,24]

Nonmetals

In addition to metals, several nonmetal components are used in implanted orthopedic devices. Bone cement can contain acrylates (used as a cement base), benzoyl peroxide (activator), antibiotics such as gentamycin, hydroquinone (acrylate stabilization) and N,N-dimethyl-p-toluidine (reaction initiator).[6] Other nonmetal components include plastics, which may be used for the plastic acetabular cup (which articulates with the metal femoral head), as well as ceramics[25,26,29]

DIAGNOSTIC TESTING IN IMPLANT HYPERSENSITIVITY REACTIONS

Diagnostic tests that can be completed or ordered include patch testing, in vitro testing, and histologic analysis of tissue. It is vital that the potential benefits, risks, and limitations of diagnostic testing are discussed with patients before completion of these tests.

Patch Testing

Patch testing is considered the best diagnostic test for IHRs.[8,20,30–32] From 2012 to 2013, Schalock and Thyssen[32] surveyed dermatologists at conferences of the ACDS (2013) and the European Society of Contact Dermatitis (ESCD) (2012) regarding their approach to metal-related IHRs. Members of these specialty groups believed that patch testing (86.1%) was more supportive of a relevant metal allergy than histology (49.6%) and in vitro testing (32.2%).

Before patch testing is completed for IHRs, it is imperative that the dermatologist and patient discuss the risks and benefits of the procedure; written informed consent is ideal. A discussion on next steps, regardless of patch test result, also should be considered, so that provider and patient expectations are in congruence. For example, the patch testing dermatologist should communicate patch test results to the patient and referring surgeon but likely would not mandate surgical removal of an implanted material; such a decision would be made by the patient and surgeon after considerations of risks and benefits of removal.

It is important for the provider to understand the type of implant and relevant components prior to patch testing for IHRs, so that the correct allergens are chosen. Several investigators have published allergens to consider in the setting of IHRs.[6,7,25,33,34] These recommended patch test series include relevant metals as well as common bone cement materials, such as acrylates, hydroquinone, benzoyl peroxide, and antibiotics.[6] In a study by Schalock and Thyssen,[35] 60% of patch testing dermatologists reported using a specialty metal series and 33% reported customizing the metals tested based on the implant. In addition, there is at least 1 commercially available metal implant series.[36] Finally, the North American Contact Dermatitis Group has designated an implant panel, which is used for all implant testing other than dental implants (Amber Reck Atwater, MD, personal communication). It also should be realized that not all allergens present in implanted materials are commercially available for purchase.

Metals in Patch Testing

Metals, as a group, are the most common contact allergens.[24] Nickel has consistently been the most prevalent allergen in North American Contact Dermatitis Group studies for years, with recent positive patch test rates between 17% and 20%.[37,38] Of note, these rates are reported mostly from referral populations, and, therefore, may overestimate rates in the general population. Other metals with high reaction frequencies in other United States–based study populations include gold, chromate, cobalt, palladium, and organic forms of mercury.[24,39,40]

Metals can cause irritant reactions, false-positive pustular reactions, or metal-specific reactions, such as the nonallergic poral reaction to cobalt and persistent reactions to gold that can last for months.[24] Certain metals, such as titanium, still lack validated standard formulations for patch testing.[27]

Concomitant positive reactions to multiple metals can occur. These usually are due to coreactivity from simultaneous exposure to multiple metals rather than cross-reactivity. Cobalt, chromium, and gold are common coreactors in patients with nickel sensitivity.[39,41] Palladium also has been found to coreact with nickel,[42] although it is not a common allergen in patients not sensitized to nickel.[39]

Metals are known to elicit delayed reactions on patch testing. In a report by the Mayo Clinic Contact Dermatitis Group, allergens with delayed positive reactions (negative readings on day 5 and positive readings on day 7) were identified.[43] The most common metals with delayed positive reactions were cobalt, palladium chloride, beryllium, potassium dicyanoaurate, and gold sodium thiosulfate. Nickel sulfate, potassium dichromate, ammonium tetrachloroplatinate, chromium (III) chloride, molybdenum, and Vitallium also had delayed positive reactions, but they were less common. For this reason, it may be prudent to complete a delayed reading in patients with suspected metal-related IHRs.

There are several studies describing higher frequencies of metal sensitivity in patients with failed implants compared with stable implants. For example, Thomas and colleagues[44] published a retrospective study of 16 patients with failed metal-on-metal hip prostheses with concomitant periprosthetic lymphocytic inflammation; 11 of 16 reacted to at least 1 metal on patch testing and 10 of 16 showed in vitro hyperreactivity to metals on the lymphocyte transformation test. Evans and colleagues[45] reported patch test results in 38 patients with stable versus failing metal implants; 9 of 14 patients with failing implants had positive patch test reactions to metals, and 0 of 24 patients with stable implants had positive patch test reactions. Frigerio and colleagues[46] described 72 patients who were patch tested both preoperatively and postoperatively. One year after implantation, 5 patients who had initially tested negative became positive for at least 1 of the metal components of their implant.

Metal Disc Patch Testing

The use of metal alloy discs, which can be affixed to the skin for testing, is not recommended for orthopedic IHR testing by the ACDS[8] or the German Implant Allergy Working Group.[20,28] Metal discs have not been evaluated in large cohorts, and the metal released from them does not simulate the peri-implant environment. In addition, there is concern for risk of irritant reactions, false-positive reactions, and false-negative reactions.[8]

In Vitro Testing

The most commonly used in vitro test for IHRs is the lymphocyte transformation test (LTT). This test, which usually is a send-out laboratory test, in theory measures lymphocyte reactivity to metals. A basic description of the LTT is as follows[47]:

1. Isolate the patient's lymphocytes from a venous blood sample.

2. Place lymphocytes in wells that are precoated with metal salts; incubate.
3. Place lymphocytes in wells with the radioactive marker [methyl-H^3]-thymidine; incubate.
4. H^3-thymidine is incorporated into DNA of dividing cells.
5. Measure H^3-thymidine radioactive uptake as counts per minute (cpm).
6. Calculate proliferation factor, or stimulation index (SI): $SI = \dfrac{cpm\ antigen\ treated\ cultures}{cpm\ control\ cultures}$
7. The threshold for a positive response is an SI > or = to 3

Niki and colleagues[48] reported a study of 92 patients who underwent 108 primary TKAs, all of whom underwent modified lymphocyte stimulation testing (mLST) to nickel, cobalt, chromium, and iron preoperatively; 24 (26%) patients had at least 1 positive response. All of the 5 patients who developed eczema postoperatively were from the mLST-positive group. Two of these had revisions of their TKA, followed by resolution of their eczema and conversion of mLST from positive to negative. Other studies report a promising correlation between metal implants and positive LTT.[44,49–52] Prospective studies are needed to examine the sensitivity of LTT, however, compared with patch testing in patients with suspected IHRs.

As discussed previously, only 32.2% of patch test specialists at contact dermatitis conferences in the United States and Europe felt that in vitro testing was supportive of a diagnosis of metal-related IHR; this test was the least supported of those included in the study.[32] Major limitations to the routine use of in vitro tests include cost, lack of availability, limitations on generalizability and applicability, lack of validation, and limited number of haptens that can be tested. The authors do not routinely use this test in the evaluation of potential metal-related IHRs.

Intradermal Testing

The 2012 to 2013 study of ACDS and ESCD member opinions asked participants to quantify their use of intradermal testing in the setting of possible metal-related IHRs.[35] A majority of respondents, 89% from ACDS and 77% from ESCD, never used intradermal testing when evaluating for IHRs. The authors do not use intradermal testing in the evaluation of potential metal-related IHRs.

Histologic Tissue Analysis

A diagnosis of cutaneous dermatitis, as expected in the setting of localized and generalized cutaneous IHRs, typically is clinical and does not require biopsy. In the setting of traditional cutaneous allergic contact dermatitis, however, it would be expected to see histology, which includes some degree of spongiotic dermatitis. Gao and colleagues[2] completed a skin biopsy for their patient with localized dermatitis from chromium IHR, and it revealed a "nonspecific perivascular lymphocytic infiltrate of the upper dermis accompanied by…eosinophils." Engelhart and Segal's[5] patient with diffuse nummular dermatitis from vanadium IHR also had a biopsy completed, and the result was "lymphoeosinophilic spongiosis." Perivascular lymphocytic infiltrates in peri-implant tissue have been interpreted by some as a marker of IHRs.[44,53] Thomas[20] argues that such a lymphocytic infiltrate represents "immunologic recognition" but not necessarily hypersensitivity. Biopsy and histologic analysis should not be used alone when making a diagnosis of IHRs.

MANAGEMENT OF IMPLANT HYPERSENSITIVITY REACTIONS
Preimplantation

Routine preimplant testing is not recommended, although it can be considered if a patient strongly believes that she or he is allergic or if requested by the referring physician.[8] Patient self-reported history of intolerance to jewelry is not historically an adequate predictor for metal allergy.[54] A more recent study noted a higher positive predictive value (71%) for the screening question, Do you have rashes when your skin is exposed to metal? and this question could be considered if metal allergy screening is desired.[55]

Even in patients who report a history of metal sensitivity or who have positive patch test reactions to metal components that are known to be present in their implants, most have no implant-related adverse events. For example, Carlsson and Moller[56] described 18 patients who did not develop any orthopedic or dermatologic complications after a mean follow-up time of 6.3 years, despite that they had positive preimplantation patch test reactions to at least 1 of the metals in their implants. Thienpont and Berger[57] reported another case of a patient with preimplant positive patch test reactions to chromium, cobalt, and nickel who accidently received a chromium-cobalt knee prosthesis due to a logistical error. The patient was followed closely and no complications were reported after 2 years of follow-up.

Atanaskova Mesinkovska and colleagues[33] published a study on implant patch testing in 2012; 31 patients completed preimplant patch testing between 2003 and 2010, and 21 of these had metal allergies. In response to this, all of the surgeons for the 21 metal-allergic patients chose an implanted device free of their allergens, and in 13 cases this required that the surgeon choose a different device than was originally planned. This study was completed in 1 institution, so it may be difficult to apply the results widely, but the positive response of surgeons to preimplant patch test results suggests that directed preimplant material choice should be possible for most patients.

One exception to the recommendation against routine preimplant patch testing is the Nuss procedure, which consists of placement of a metal bar in the chest for correction of severe pectus excavatum deformity. The ACDS recommends preimplant testing prior to the Nuss procedure,[8] and this is in part based on retrospective surgical studies that document higher-than-expected clinical symptoms or metal allergy.[58] Obermeyer and colleagues,[59] a group of surgeons who perform the Nuss procedure, recently published an update: allergy frequency was low, with similar rates regardless of whether preimplant testing was selective (personal or family history of metal hypersensitivity) or routine (test everyone). They highlighted the concept that if selective preimplant testing is preferred, it should be completed for patients with a personal or family history of metal sensitivity and for female patients, because these groups were at higher risk for IHRs.

Postimplantation

Contact dermatitis and patch test specialists often have individual opinions on when postimplant patch testing should be completed, in part because of the controversy over which presentations are the most relevant. The authors tend to complete postimplant patch testing when there is localized peri-implant dermatitis, there is generalized dermatitis with a timeline that is consistent with an implant source, or requested by a referring surgeon.

There are data on how contact dermatitis and patch test specialists approach postimplant patch testing. Schalock and Thyssen[32] asked attendees of the 24th annual meeting of the ACDS (2013) and the 11th congress of the ESCD (2012) the following question: When evaluating a patient with a suspected hypersensitivity reaction following device implant, what do you feel is supportive of a relevant metal allergy? Possible responses were based on criteria previously proposed by Thyssen and colleagues[25] in 2011. Based on the results of this study, the diagnostic criteria for IHRs were refined as follows:

Major criteria

1. Eruption overlying the metal implant

2. Positive patch test reaction to a metal used in the implant
3. Complete recovery after removal of the offending implant
4. Chronic dermatitis beginning weeks to months after metallic implantation

Minor criteria

1. Therapy-resistant dermatitis
2. Morphology consistent with dermatitis (erythema, induration, papules, vesicles)
3. Systemic allergic dermatitis reaction
4. Histology consistent with allergic contact dermatitis
5. Positive in vitro test to metals, for example, the lymphocyte transformation test

These criteria were organized based on the percentage of overall respondents who agreed that they were supportive of a relevant allergy, with 78.3% and above supportive of the major criteria and 60.9% and below in support of the minor criteria. There is no designated point system for determining relevance of potential IHRs, and the criteria have not yet been validated. These major and minor criteria are a starting point for making a decision about whether IHRs are present.

Atanaskova Mesinkovska and colleagues'[33] 2012 study on implant patch testing also included postimplant patients; 41 patients completed postimplant patch testing between 2003 and 2010; 15 patients had metal positive patch test reactions, but only 10 of these (24%) had relevant metal positive patch test reactions, with nickel the most common; 6 patients with relevant positive patch test reactions had their implant removed, and their symptoms resolved. The 4 patients with relevant reactions who did not have their implants removed had persistent symptoms. These data suggest that implanted device revision should be considered in the setting of symptomatic IHRs with relevant metal positive patch test reactions.

Clinical Relevance

Determining the clinical relevance in individual cases can be complicated by several factors, including the following:

1. Metal hypersensitivity is common, with nickel the most common positive patch test reaction in referral populations.
2. Positive patch test reactions not always are clinically relevant.
3. Postoperative pain and other implant-related complications are not uncommon, and causes are various, including aseptic osteolysis, infection, recurrent dislocation, and fractures.

4. The only way to definitively confirm that implant-related complications are due to IHRs is to remove the device and monitor for clinical improvement.

SUMMARY

Orthopedic IHRs are uncommon and can be devastating for patients. It is vital for dermatologists and surgeons to be aware of the potential clinical presentations of IHRs and to evaluate and manage affected patients appropriately. Progress has been made in the understanding of IHRs, but more research is needed.

CONFLICT OF INTEREST

M.B. Innes: none. A.R. Atwater: A.R. Atwater received a Pfizer Independent Grant for Learning and Change.

REFERENCES

1. Thomas P, Gollwitzer H, Maier S, et al. Osteosynthesis associated contact dermatitis with unusual perpetuation of hyperreactivity in a nickel allergic patient. Contact Dermatitis 2006;54(4):222–5.
2. Gao X, He RX, Yan SG, et al. Dermatitis associated with chromium following total knee arthroplasty. J Arthroplasty 2011;26(4):665.e13-6.
3. Treudler R, Simon JC. Benzoyl peroxide: is it a relevant bone cement allergen in patients with orthopaedic implants? Contact Dermatitis 2007;57(3):177–80.
4. Barranco VP, Soloman H. Eczematous dermatitis from nickel. JAMA 1972;220(9):1244.
5. Engelhart S, Segal RJ. Allergic reaction to vanadium causes a diffuse eczematous eruption and titanium alloy orthopedic implant failure. Cutis 2017;99(4):245–9.
6. Basko-Plluska JL, Thyssen JP, Schalock PC. Cutaneous and systemic hypersensitivity reactions to metallic implants. Dermatitis 2011;22(2):65–79.
7. Schalock PC, Menne T, Johansen JD, et al. Hypersensitivity reactions to metallic implants - diagnostic algorithm and suggested patch test series for clinical use. Contact Dermatitis 2012;66(1):4–19.
8. Schalock PC, Crawford G, Nedorost S, et al. Patch testing for evaluation of hypersensitivity to implanted metal devices: a perspective from the American Contact Dermatitis Society. Dermatitis 2016;27(5):241–7.
9. Christiansen RJ, Münch HJ, Bonefeld CM, et al. Cytokine Profile in Patients with Aseptic Loosening of Total Hip Replacements and Its Relation to Metal Release and Metal Allergy. J Clin Med 2019;8(8):1259.

10. Holt G, Murnaghan C, Reilly J, et al. The biology of aseptic osteolysis. Clin Orthop Relat Res 2007;460: 240–52.

11. Brodner W, Bitzan P, Meisinger V, et al. Elevated serum cobalt with metal-on-metal articulating surfaces. J Bone Joint Surg Br 1997;79(2):316–21.

12. Brodner W, Bitzan P, Meisinger V, et al. Serum cobalt levels after metal-on-metal total hip arthroplasty. J Bone Joint Surg Am 2003;85(11):2168–73.

13. Schaffer AW, Pilger A, Engelhardt C, et al. Increased blood cobalt and chromium after total hip replacement. J Toxicol Clin Toxicol 1999;37(7):839–44.

14. Hallab NJ, Anderson S, Caicedo M, et al. Immune responses correlate with serum-metal in metal-on-metal hip arthroplasty. J Arthroplasty 2004;19(8 Suppl 3):88–93.

15. Jacobs JJ, Urban RM, Hallab NJ, et al. Metal-on-metal bearing surfaces. J Am Acad Orthop Surg 2009;17(2):69–76.

16. Okazaki Y, Gotoh E. Comparison of metal release from various metallic biomaterials in vitro. Biomaterials 2005;26(1):11–21.

17. Savarino L, Tigani D, Greco M, et al. The potential role of metal ion release as a marker of loosening in patients with total knee replacement: a cohort study. J Bone Joint Surg Br 2010;92(5):634–8.

18. Lass R, Grubl A, Kolb A, et al. Comparison of synovial fluid, urine, and serum ion levels in metal-on-metal total hip arthroplasty at a minimum follow-up of 18 years. J Orthop Res 2014;32(9):1234–40.

19. Case CP, Langkamer VG, James C, et al. Widespread dissemination of metal debris from implants. J Bone Joint Surg Br 1994;76(5):701–12.

20. Thomas P. Patch testing and hypersensitivity reactions to metallic implants: still many open questions. Dermatitis 2013;24(3):106–7.

21. Crawford GH. The role of patch testing in the evaluation of orthopedic implant-related adverse effects: current evidence does not support broad use. Dermatitis 2013;24(3):99–103.

22. Gallo J, Goodman SB, Konttinen YT, et al. Particle disease: biologic mechanisms of periprosthetic osteolysis in total hip arthroplasty. Innate Immun 2013;19(2):213–24.

23. Gallo J, Vaculova J, Goodman SB, et al. Contributions of human tissue analysis to understanding the mechanisms of loosening and osteolysis in total hip replacement. Acta Biomater 2014;10(6): 2354–66.

24. Fisher AA, Fowler JF, Zirwas MJ, et al. Fisher's contact dermatitis. 7th edition. Phoenix (AZ): Contact Dermatitis Institute; 2019.

25. Thyssen JP, Menne T, Schalock PC, et al. Pragmatic approach to the clinical work-up of patients with putative allergic disease to metallic orthopaedic implants before and after surgery. Br J Dermatol 2011;164(3):473–8.

26. Nasab MBN, Hassan MR. Metallic biomaterials of knee and hip-a review. Trends Biomater Artif Organs 2010;24(1):69–82.

27. Wood MM, Warshaw EM. Hypersensitivity reactions to titanium: diagnosis and management. Dermatitis 2015;26(1):7–25.

28. Thomas P, Schuh A, Ring J, et al. Orthopedic surgical implants and allergies: joint statement by the implant allergy working group (AK 20) of the DGOOC (German association of orthopedics and orthopedic surgery), DKG (German contact dermatitis research group) and dgaki (German society for allergology and clinical immunology). Orthopade 2008;37(1):75–88.

29. Navarro M, Michiardi A, Castano O, et al. Biomaterials in orthopaedics. J R Soc Interface 2008;5(27): 1137–58.

30. Schalock PC. Pragmatism and the evaluation of metal hypersensitivity reactions. Dermatitis 2013; 24(3):104–5.

31. Honari G, Taylor JS. Commentary on Crawford, et al, The role of patch testing in the evaluation of orthopedic implant-related adverse effects: current evidence does not support broad use. Dermatitis 2013;24(3):108–11.

32. Schalock PC, Thyssen JP. Patch testers' opinions regarding diagnostic criteria for metal hypersensitivity reactions to metallic implants. Dermatitis 2013; 24(4):183–5.

33. Atanaskova Mesinkovska N, Tellez A, Molina L, et al. The effect of patch testing on surgical practices and outcomes in orthopedic patients with metal implants. Arch Dermatol 2012;148(6):687–93.

34. Reed KB, Davis MDP, Nakamura K, et al. Retrospective Evaluation of Patch Testing Before or After Metal Device Implantation. Arch Dermatol 2008;144(8): 999–1007.

35. Schalock PC, Thyssen JP. Metal hypersensitivity reactions to implants: opinions and practices of patch testing dermatologists. Dermatitis 2013;24(6): 313–20.

36. Available at: https://www.smartpracticecanada.com/shop/wa/style?id=SCSERIESOINA. Accessed September 15, 2019.

37. DeKoven JG, Warshaw EM, Belsito DV, et al. North American Contact Dermatitis Group Patch Test Results 2013-2014. Dermatitis 2017;28(1):33–46.

38. DeKoven JG, Warshaw EM, Zug KA, et al. North American Contact Dermatitis Group Patch Test Results: 2015-2016. Dermatitis 2018;29(6):297–309.

39. Rastogi S, Patel KR, Singam V, et al. Associations of Nickel Co-Reactions and Metal Polysensitization in Adults. Dermatitis 2018;29(6):316–20.

40. Davis MD, Wang MZ, Yiannias JA, et al. Patch testing with a large series of metal allergens: findings from more than 1,000 patients in one decade at Mayo Clinic. Dermatitis 2011;22(5):256–71.

41. Duarte I, Mendonca RF, Korkes KL, et al. Nickel, chromium and cobalt: the relevant allergens in allergic contact dermatitis. Comparative study between two periods: 1995-2002 and 2003-2015. An Bras Dermatol 2018;93(1):59–62.

42. Durosaro O, el-Azhary RA. A 10-year retrospective study on palladium sensitivity. Dermatitis 2009; 20(4):208–13.

43. Chaudhry HM, Drage LA, El-Azhary RA, et al. Delayed patch-test reading after 5 days: an update from the Mayo Clinic Contact Dermatitis Group. Dermatitis 2017;28(4):253–60.

44. Thomas P, Braathen LR, Dorig M, et al. Increased metal allergy in patients with failed metal-on-metal hip arthroplasty and peri-implant T-lymphocytic inflammation. Allergy 2009;64(8):1157–65.

45. Evans EM, Freeman MA, Miller AJ, et al. Metal sensitivity as a cause of bone necrosis and loosening of the prosthesis in total joint replacement. J Bone Joint Surg Br 1974;56-b(4):626–42.

46. Frigerio E, Pigatto PD, Guzzi G, et al. Metal sensitivity in patients with orthopaedic implants: a prospective study. Contact Dermatitis 2011;64(5): 273–9.

47. Stejskal VD, Cederbrant K, Lindvall A, et al. MELISA-an in vitro tool for the study of metal allergy. Toxicol In Vitro 1994;8(5):991–1000.

48. Niki Y, Matsumoto H, Otani T, et al. Screening for symptomatic metal sensitivity: a prospective study of 92 patients undergoing total knee arthroplasty. Biomaterials 2005;26(9):1019–26.

49. Thomas P, von der Helm C, Schopf C, et al. Patients with intolerance reactions to total knee replacement: combined assessment of allergy diagnostics, peri-prosthetic histology, and peri-implant cytokine expression pattern. Biomed Res Int 2015;2015: 910156.

50. Everness KM, Gawkrodger DJ, Botham PA, et al. The discrimination between nickel-sensitive and non-nickel-sensitive subjects by an in vitro lymphocyte transformation test. Br J Dermatol 1990; 122(3):293–8.

51. Svejgaard E, Morling N, Svejgaard A, et al. Lymphocyte transformation induced by nickel sulphate: an in vitro study of subjects with and without a positive nickel patch test. Acta Derm Venereol 1978;58(3): 245–50.

52. Veien NK, Svejgaard E. Lymphocyte transformation in patients with cobalt dermatitis. Br J Dermatol 1978;99(2):191–6.

53. Krenn V, Morawietz L, Perino G, et al. Revised histopathological consensus classification of joint implant related pathology. Pathol Res Pract 2014;210(12): 779–86.

54. Josefson A, Färm G, Meding B. Validity of self-reported nickel allergy. Contact Dermatitis 2010; 62(5):289–93.

55. Ko LN, Kroshinsky D, Schalock PC. Assessing the validity of self-reported history of rash caused by metal or jewellery. Contact Dermatitis 2018;78(3): 208–10.

56. Carlsson A, Moller H. Implantation of orthopaedic devices in patients with metal allergy. Acta Derm Venereol 1989;69(1):62–6.

57. Thienpont E, Berger Y. No allergic reaction after TKA in a chrome-cobalt-nickel-sensitive patient: case report and review of the literature. Knee Surg Sports Traumatol Arthrosc 2013;21(3):636–40.

58. Shah B, Cohee A, Deyerle A, et al. High rates of metal allergy amongst Nuss procedure patients dictate broader pre-operative testing. J Pediatr Surg 2014;49(3):451–4.

59. Obermeyer RJ, Gaffar S, Kelly REJ, et al. Selective versus routine patch metal allergy testing to select bar material for the Nuss procedure in 932 patients over 10 years. J Pediatr Surg 2018;53(2):260–4.

Allergic Contact Dermatitis to Fragrances

Margo J. Reeder, MD

KEYWORDS

- Fragrance • Perfume • Allergic contact dermatitis • Essential oils • Botanicals

KEY POINTS

- Allergic contact dermatitis to fragrance is common, and positive reaction rates range from 5% to 11% in patch-test populations.
- Fragrance allergy is more common in women and can present with dermatitis on the face, eyelids, hands, or generalized.
- Supplementing fragrance screeners with additional fragrance chemicals can increase the diagnostic yield for detecting allergic contact dermatitis.

INTRODUCTION

Allergic contact dermatitis (ACD) to fragrances remains a common cause of allergy. Patients are exposed to fragrances through personal care products, cleaning products, and aromatherapy. The popular trend of essential oils continues to sensitize patients to fragrances. This review summarizes ACD to fragrances, including positive reaction rates on patch testing, site-specific dermatitis related to fragrances, essential oils, botanical ingredients, and challenges for the fragrance-allergic patient.

CONTACT DERMATITIS TO FRAGRANCES

Fragrances are chemicals added to products with the usual intention of providing a pleasant scent. Fragrances can be encountered in all types of personal care products, such as shampoos, soaps, lotions, makeup, and sunscreens. Fragrances can also be added to products to mask an unpleasant scent, and they may be added to cleaning chemicals or industrial chemicals. The use of masking fragrances is common in cleaning and industrial chemicals. Paper products, detergents, and medical products frequently contain additive fragrances. In 2017, fragrance global sales topped

$8.2 billion, excluding sales in the United States and Canada.[1] The fragrance industry also contributes 415,000 jobs to the workplace.[1]

Fragrances can be characterized as natural or synthetic. Natural fragrances are derived from organic materials, including plants and flowers. Essential oils and botanicals are an example of natural fragrances. Synthetic fragrances are those created in a laboratory and may be produced to mimic a natural fragrance while using less organic resources.[2]

Fragrance can cause both allergic and irritant dermatitis. Irritant dermatitis from fragrances is commonly seen in patients with atopic diathesis. In general, patients with active dermatitis or a history of "sensitive skin" are commonly advised to avoid fragrances in care products, and patients may seek out products that are labeled as "fragrance free." This review focuses on fragrance allergy.

EPIDEMIOLOGY OF FRAGRANCE ALLERGY

ACD from fragrances is common. In the general population, the allergic reaction rate to fragrances varies between 0.7% and 2.6%.[3] A cross-sectional study of 5 European countries found the prevalence of fragrance allergy is 1.9% to

Department of Dermatology, University of Wisconsin School of Medicine and Public Health, 1 South Park Street, 7th Floor, Madison, WI 53715, USA
E-mail address: mreeder@dermatology.wisc.edu

Dermatol Clin 38 (2020) 371–377
https://doi.org/10.1016/j.det.2020.02.009
0733-8635/20/© 2020 Elsevier Inc. All rights reserved.

2.6% among the general population.[4] However, the rate of contact allergy to fragrances is much higher in a referral-based population. In the North American Contact Dermatitis Group (NACDG) 2015 to 2016 cycle, fragrances were among the top positive allergens. Fragrance mix 1 (FM1), Fragrance mix 2 (FM2) (components are listed in **Table 1**), and Balsam of Peru are considered markers for fragrance allergy, and reaction rates range from 5.3% to 11.3%.[5] Positive reaction rates from recent NACDG cycles to common fragrance chemicals are listed in **Table 2**.[5] However, patch testing with FM1, FM2, and Balsam of Peru alone will not detect all fragrance-allergic patients. Fragrance chemicals are often added to baseline series in order to better detect fragrance allergy. Hydroxyisohexyl 3-cyclohexene carboxaldehyde (HICC) is the most common allergen in FM2, and positive reaction rates to HICC range from 1.5% to 3%. HICC alone was recommended to be added to the European Baseline Series in 2008.[6]

ACD to fragrances is more commonly seen in female patients with women being 1.3 times more likely to be allergic to fragrances than men.[7] In general, most large patch test studies have more women than men. Despite the female predominance in studies, fragrance allergies tend to still disproportionately affect women, perhaps because of increased use of cosmetics and perfumed products. Women allergic to fragrances are most commonly in their 40s, whereas men allergic to fragrances tend to be 5 to 6 years older.[7]

Fragrance allergy can be associated with all sites of dermatitis. An analysis from the European Surveillance System on Contact Allergies found that positive reactions to fragrance were associated with all specific sites of dermatitis excluding the feet.[8] Fragrance allergy has also been frequently associated with hand dermatitis. A cross-sectional analysis of NACDG data from 1994 to 2004 found that of patch tested patients with allergic hand dermatitis, 11.3% were positive to fragrance mix and 9.6% were positive to Balsam of Peru.[9] Other common allergens included nickel, preservatives, rubber, and antibiotics.[9]

Eyelid dermatitis is another site where ACD to fragrances is a common culprit. For the eyelids, the exposure can be direct contact (such as products applied to the hair or eyelids) and airborne contact (including mists, sprays, and aerosols). Fragrances are a common cause of eyelid dermatitis. In a single-center review of 100 consecutive patients patch tested for eyelid dermatitis, 42% were positive to one or more fragrance chemical.[10]

Fragrances may also be a source for occupational dermatitis. Of reported occupational skin disease in the United Kingdom between 1996 and 2015, 6% were related to fragrance allergy and were more commonly reported in women. Hairdressers and beauticians were particularly at risk, followed by therapists (including aromatherapists) and those in the food preparation industry.[11] Fragrances in the workplace may also be from exposure to essential oils. Diffusers are more commonly used in shared office spaces and represent an important exposure. Diffusion of essential oils can cause an airborne contact dermatitis leading to rash on exposed skin, such as the eyelids, face, and hands. Other important occupation exposures include the addition of masking fragrances to strongly scented chemicals. Fragrances are still added to industrial chemicals, metalworking fluids, and cleaning chemicals with the purpose of masking an unpleasant odor.

DETECTING FRAGRANCE ALLERGY

Patch testing with too few fragrance chemicals may also miss fragrance-allergic patients. FM1, FM2, and Balsam of Peru are considered the fragrance screening chemicals that are found on

Table 1 Components of fragrance mixes commonly found in a standard tray of allergens	
FM1, 8.0% petrolatum*	Cinnamyl alcohol 1% pet Cinnamal 1% pet Hydroxycitronellal 1% pet Amyl cinnamal 1% pet Geraniol 1% pet Eugenol 1% pet Isoeugenol 1% pet Oakmoss Absolute 1% pet *Contains 5% sorbitan sesquioleate as emulsifier
FM2, 14% petrolatum	Hexyl cinnamic aldehyde 5% pet Hydroxyisohexyl 3-cyclohexene carboxaldehyde 2.5% pet Farnesol 2.5% pet Coumarin 2.5% pet Citral 1% pet Citronellol 0.5% pet

Table 2
Positive reaction rates based on previous North American Contact Dermatitis Group cycles

Allergen	N	2015–2016 (%)	2013–2014 (%)	2011–2012 (%)
FM1, 8.0% petrolatum	5595	11.3	11.9	12.1
FM2, 14% petrolatum	5594	5.3	5.7	5.2
Balsam of Peru, 25% petrolatum	5595	7.0	7.2	7.9
Ylang ylang oil, 2.0% petrolatum	5594	1.3	1.2	0.7
Melaleuca alternifoilia (tea tree leaf oil), oxidized 5.0% petrolatum	5593	1.2	0.9	0.8
Mentha piperita oil (peppermint oil) 2.0% petrolatum	5591	0.6	0.6	0.4
Lavandula angustifolia oil (lavender oil), 2.0% petrolatum	5594	0.5	0.3	0.4

Data from DeKoven JG, Warshaw EM, Zug KA, et al. North American Contact Dermatitis Group Patch Test Results: 2015-2016. Dermatitis 2018;29(6):297-309.

most standard trays. However, patch testing with just these 3 chemicals can miss a significant number of fragrance-allergic patients. In a population of 1951 eczema patients who underwent patch testing with a standard and a fragrance tray, 14.4% (281 patients) were allergic to a fragrance. However, only 57.6% (117 patients) reacted to a fragrance in the screening series, meaning that 42.4% of patients would have been missed if the supplemental tray was not added. The most commonly positive individual fragrances were cinnamyl alcohol, Evernia furfuracea, isoeugenol, Evernia prunastri, and cinnamal.[12]

Patch testing with limonene and linalool further increases the ability to diagnose fragrance allergy. In a study of 821 consecutively patch tested patients, 9.4% were positive to hydroperoxide of limonene and 11.7% were positive to linalool.[13] Of all the fragrance-allergic patients in this series, 10% were positive to limonene and/or linalool but were negative to a fragrance marker on the standard series.[13] In another single-institution study of 103 patients who were tested to linalool, hydroperoxides of linalool, D-limonene, and/or hydroperoxides of D-limonene, 19% were positive to hydroperoxides of limonene and 7% were positive to hydroperoxides of linalool. Importantly, very few patients reacted to linalool (10%), and no patients were positive to D-limonene.[14] This finding suggests that patch testing with the hydroperoxides of limonene and hydroperoxides of linalool is important in suspected fragrance-allergic patients.

Patients allergic to essential oils may also be missed if expanded patch testing is not

performed. In a study of 62,354 patch-test patients from North America and Europe, 1.4% (854) of patients reacted to an essential oil but were negative to a fragrance marker.[15] For the patients from North America, Melaluca (tea tree) and ylang ylang were common essential oils that would have been missed by testing with fragrance markers alone.[15]

PATCH TESTING PITFALLS: TECHNIQUE

Fragrances are volatile chemicals and are prone to degradation. A potential pitfall in patch testing, false negative reactions to fragrances may occur if trays are assembled ahead of time because allergens may evaporate and degrade over time.[16,17] Instead, fragrance allergens should be assembled on chambers directly before application to the patient. Patch test reactions to fragrances can also peak earlier than other allergens. Often, fragrance chemicals can elicit a positive reaction at the 48-hour reading.[18] Delayed reactions done at 120 hours or later may start to see a decline in the degree of positive reactivity, and weak positive reactions may be missed if a delayed reading is done only at 144 hours.

Differences also exist in the ability to detect fragrance allergy between patch testing systems. The TRUE test is a preloaded Food and Drug Administration–approved commercially available patch test system that screens for 35 common allergens plus a negative control.[19] Although the TRUE test can be an initial screen, it fails to detect allergies in 25% to 40% of patients.[5] In the chamber method, individual allergens are loaded into either plastic or metal chambers and fixed to the patient. Greater ability to customize allergens to the patient's dermatitis exists with the chamber method. The chamber method is used by the NACDG and the International Contact Dermatitis Research Group.

The TRUE test may fail to detect patients with fragrance allergies. In a comparative study of the TRUE test versus chamber method, the TRUE test failed to detect 50% of positive reactions to fragrance.[20] Balsam of Peru in particular is frequently missed by TRUE testing.[21] However, a larger study examining FM1 reactions compared with the TRUE test showed that although chamber method produced more positive reactions, the reactions found with the TRUE test had a larger percent of clinical relevance, calling for careful interpretation of weak positive reactions to fragrances on chamber method.[22]

ESSENTIAL OILS

The use of essential oils represents a popular trend, which is also exposing numerous patients to concentrated chemicals known to elicit ACD. Essential oils are often seen by the public as a safe alternative to traditional medicine. Dermatologists likely encounter the use of essential oils when they are used for medicinal purposes or aromatherapy. Many essential oils have purported health benefits, such as cleansing, detoxifying, awakening, and healing. However, essential oils have long been known to cause ACD. Many different methods of using essential oils are available. Diffusing oils into the air in a mist is popular for bedrooms and home use, but increasingly, diffusers may also be spotted at gyms and daycare centers. Essential oils may also be applied directly to the skin, either diluted in carrier oil or "as is." Many essential oil companies warn of the sensitizing nature of essential oils given their high concentration, but consumers may not follow these recommendations. Information found on essential oil manufacturer Web sites can be misleading for consumers, particularly statements that rashes from essential oils may be from "detoxification" and not contact dermatitis.[23] Essential oils are sometimes added to laundry or cosmetics and even may be ingested for dubious health benefits. Aside from cosmetic use, essential oils may also be used as a flavoring for various foods, including beverages, spices, and food preservation. Essential oils may be added to different household products in place of other fragrances.[24]

Most essential oils are created by the process of steam distillation. Essential oils that are citrus are derived from the fruit peels of orange, lime, lemon, or tangerine through a mechanical cold press.[25] Although essential oils are often marketed as "pure," the plant-derived nature of essential oils means that the oils can often contain hundreds of different compounds. Most essential oils upon mass spectrometry analysis contain between 100 and 250 different chemicals, but some oils contain up to 500 different chemicals.[26] The variation in different batches of essential oils can be related to the crop of plant or fruit, storage, temperature, and factors related to the products and production.[26] Certain chemical components have been found to be dominant in essential oils. Limonene is found in nearly all citrus-related oils. Anethole is found in most aniseed oils and eugenol is found in 90% of clove oils. Other chemicals found in greater than 90% of essential oils include caryophyllene, pinene, terpineol, cadinene, and myrcene.[26]

More than 80 essential oils have been described in the literature as causes of ACD. The most common essential oils known to cause ACD include tea tree, turpentine, orange, citronella, ylang ylang, sandalwood, and clove.[27] Currently, the NACDG includes 3 essential oils on the screening tray: tea tree, ylang ylang, and peppermint. These essential oils are in addition to FM1, FM2, Balsam of Peru, hydroperoxides of limonene, and hydroperoxides and linalool. Most patch testing hapten companies have essential oil allergens available for purchase for supplementing a standard tray of chemicals.

NATURAL INGREDIENTS

Similar to essential oils, natural or botanical ingredients are commonly found in cosmetic products and represent a potential source of exposure for fragrance-allergic patients. Plant-derived ingredients are often used instead of fragrances. Ingredients such as aloe vera, chamomile, arnica, calendula, echinacea, and other plants are increasingly added to personal care products. Patients often gravitate toward products that contain natural ingredients because of a perceived safety associated with natural over synthetic ingredients. A survey of 1274 users of botanical products cited reasons for using natural products as curiosity (52%), perceived safety (38%), failure of conventional therapy (7%), and mistrust in traditional topical products (3%).[28] Medicinal uses of natural products included moisturization, skin cleansing, itching, eczema, and antiaging among others.[28]

In one retrospective study of 125[29] patients with contact allergy to an herbal preparation, most patients were using the natural product to treat another medical condition. Eczema, leg ulcers, wounds, and moisturizers were common conditions that led to the use of botanical products. Implicated allergens included Balsam of Peru, compositae family plants, and tincture of benzoin.[29]

Products containing many botanical and plant-derived ingredients may frequently be listed as "fragrance-free," which is confusing for the consumer. These "natural" labeled products can still lead to ACD for some fragrance-allergic patients and should be avoided. Botanical allergic patients should be certain to avoid related botanical ingredients in personal care products. In a study of 12 patients with known allergies to either chamomile or arnica on previous patch testing, 8/12 of the chamomile allergic and 5/6 of the arnica allergic reacted to botanical-containing products, respectively.[30] The implications of natural ingredients for fragrance-allergic patients remain unclear. In general, avoidance of fragrances includes botanical ingredients. When in doubt, a repeat open application test is helpful. In this test, the product should be applied below the crease of the arm twice daily for 2 to 4 weeks. If a reaction does not occur, the product will likely be tolerated. Importantly, with fragrance-allergic patients, it has been shown that the repeat open application test must be done for up to 4 weeks to elicit a positive reaction.[31]

CHALLENGES FOR THE FRAGRANCE-ALLERGIC PATIENT

A unique challenge that fragrance-allergic patients face in safe product selection primarily has to do with regulations on fragrance labeling in the United States. Fragrances are considered a "trade secret," and individual components need not be fully disclosed on the ingredient label.[32] In order to avoid all potential exposure to a fragrance ingredient, patients must choose products that are free of fragrances. Finding fragrance-free products is challenging given the ubiquitous nature of fragrances as well as the use of masking fragrances in cosmetics. Products labeled as "unscented" may lead to inadvertent exposure to fragrances given the product could contain a masking fragrance to mask an unpleasant odor. To contrast, in the European Union, the top 26 fragrance chemicals known to cause ACD must be labeled on products (**Box 1**).[33]

Because ingredients are characterized by their function in the product, patients may also be inadvertently exposed to fragrances in a product that is listed as "fragrance free." For example, benzyl alcohol functions as a fragrance as well as a preservative. If it is used in a product as a preservative (and not a fragrance), the company may list the ingredient

---

Box 1
List of 26 fragrances that must be includes on labels in European Union

Amyl cinnamal
Amyl cinnamyl alcohol
Benzyl alcohol
Benzyl salicylate
Cinnamyl alcohol
Cinnamal
Citral
Coumarin
Eugenol
Geraniol
Hydroxycitronellal
Hydroxymethylpentyl-cyclohexenecarboxaldehyde
Isoeugenol
Anisyl alcohol
Benzyl benzoate
Benzyl cinnamate
Citronellol
Farnesol
Hexyl cinnamaldehyde
Lilial
D-Limonene
Linalool
Methyl heptine carbonate
3-Methyl-4-(2,6,6-trimethyl-2-cyclohexen-1-yl)-3-buten-2-one
Oak moss
Tree moss

Adapted from Scientific Committee on Consumer Safety (SCCS). Opinion on Fragrance allergens in cosmetic products. Brussels: European Union; 2011; with permission.

---

yet still label the product as fragrance free. A recent review found that 45% (18/40) of best-selling moisturizers listed as "fragrance free" actually contained a fragrance or botanical cross-reactor.[34]

Hair care products in general contain a significant amount of fragrances. A recent query of the American Contact Dermatitis Society Contact Allergy Management Program (CAMP) found that of the 306 shampoos listed in CAMP, only 16 were fragrance free. For styling products, only 2.8% (9/324) were free of fragrances.[35] Education on label reading as well as access to patient resources can greatly help those diagnosed with ACD to fragrances.

SUMMARY

ACD to fragrances is common and is seen in 5% to 15% of patch tested patients. Patients are exposed to fragrances through both household and personal care products. Fragrance allergy commonly presents on the face, eyelids, and hands, but other sites may be affected. Although patch testing with FM1, FM2, and Balsam of Peru will screen for fragrance allergy, the diagnostic yield is improved by the addition of the hydroperoxides of linalool, hydroperoxides of limonene, and HICC. The popularity of essential oils represents an important source of fragrance allergy. The increasingly common use of botanicals in personal care products and incomplete fragrance labeling by companies leads to additional challenges for the fragrance-allergic patient.

DISCLOSURE

Nothing to disclose.

REFERENCES

1. The International Fragrance Association. The value of fragrance. A socio-economic contribution study for the global fragrance industry. Available at: https://ifrafragrance.org/docs/default-source/policy-documents/pwc-value-of-fragrance-report-2019.pdf?sfvrsn=b3d049c8_0. Accessed July 11 2019.
2. The International Fragrance Association. What is a fragrance?. Available at: https://ifrafragrance.org/what-we-do/what-is-a-fragrance. Accessed August 15, 2019.
3. Bruze M, Mowitz M, Ofenloch R, et al. The significance of batch and patch test method in establishing contact allergy to fragrance mix I EDEN Fragrance Study Group. Contact Dermatitis 2019; 81:104–9.
4. Diepgen T, Ofenloch R, Bruze M, et al. Prevalence of fragrance contact allergy in the general population of five European countries: a cross-sectional study. Br J Dermatol 2015;173:1411–9.
5. DeKoven JG, Warshaw EM, Zug KA, et al. North American Contact Dermatitis Group patch test results: 2015-2016. Dermatitis 2018;29(6):297–309.
6. Bruze M, Andersen KE, Goossens A, on behalf of the ESCD and EECDRG. Recommendation to include fragrance mix 2 and hydroxyisohexyl 3-cyclohexene carboxaldehyde (Lyral) in the European baseline patch test series. Contact Dermatitis 2008;58:129–33.
7. Buckley D, Wakelin S, Seed P, et al. The frequency of fragrance allergy in a patch-test population over a 17-year period. Br J Dermatol 2000;142(2): 279–83.
8. Oosterhaven JAF, Uter W, Aberer W, et al. European Surveillance System on Contact Allergies (ESSCA): contact allergies in relation to body sites in patients with allergic contact dermatitis. Contact Dermatitis 2019;80:263–72.
9. Warshaw EM, Ahmed RL, Belsito DV, et al. Contact dermatitis of the hands: cross-sectional analyses of North American Contact Dermatitis Group data, 1994-2004. J Am Acad Dermatol 2007;57: 301–14.
10. Wenk KS, Ehrlich A. Fragrance series testing in eyelid dermatitis. Dermatitis 2012;23(1):22–6.
11. Montgomery RL, Agius R, Wilkinson SM, et al. UK trends of allergic occupational skin disease attributed to fragrances 1996–2015. Contact Dermatitis 2018;78(1):33–40.
12. Mann J, McFadden JP, White JM, et al. Baseline series fragrance markers fail to predict contact allergy. Contact Dermatitis 2014;70(5):276–81.
13. Dittmar D, Schuttelaar MLA. Contact sensitization to hydroperoxides of limonene and linalool: results of consecutive patch testing and clinical relevance. Contact Dermatitis 2019;80(2):101–9.
14. Nath NS, Liu B, Green C, et al. Contact allergy to hydroperoxides of linalool and D-limonene in a US population. Dermatitis 2017;28(5):313–6.
15. Warshaw EM, Zug KA, Belsito DV, et al. Positive patch-test reactions to essential oils in consecutive patients from North America and Central Europe. Dermatitis 2017;28(4):246–52.
16. Mowitz M, Zimerson E, Svedman C, et al. Stability of fragrance patch test preparations applied in test chambers. Br J Dermatol 2012;167(4): 822–7.
17. Hamann D, Hamann CR, Zimerson E, et al. Hydroxyisohexyl 3-cyclohexene carboxaldehyde (Lyral) in patch test preparations under varied storage conditions. Dermatitis 2013;24(5):246–8.
18. Shehade S, Beck M, Hillier V. Epidemiological survey of standard series patch test results and observations on day 2 and day 4 readings. Contact Dermatitis 1991;24(2):119–22.
19. Smart practice. Available at: https://www.smartpractice.com/shop/wa/category?cn=T.R.U.E.-TEST®-Ready-to-Use-Patch-Test-Panels&id=508222&m=SPA. Accessed August 15, 2019.
20. Suneja T, Belsito DV. Comparative study of Finn chambers and T.R.U.E. test methodologies in detecting the relevant allergens inducing contact dermatitis. J Am Acad Dermatol 2001;45: 836–9.
21. Lazarov A, David M, Abraham D, et al. Comparison of reactivity to allergens using the True test and IQ chamber system. Contact Dermatitis 2007;56: 140–5.

22. Mortz CG, Andersen KE. Fragrance mix I patch test reactions in 5006 consecutive dermatitis patients tested with True Test® and Trolab® test material. Contact Dermatitis 2010;63:248–53.

23. Essential oil safety guide. Available at: https://www.youngliving.com/en_US/discover/essential-oil-safety. Accessed August 8, 2019.

24. de Groot AC, Schmidt E. Essential oils: contact allergy and chemical composition. II. General aspects of essential oils. Dermatitis 2016;27:43–9.

25. deGroot AC, Schmidt E. Essential oils, part I: introduction. Dermatitis 2016;27(2):39–42.

26. de Groot AC, Schmidt E. Essential oils: contact allergy and chemical composition. III. Chemical composition. Dermatitis 2016;27:161–9.

27. de Groot AC, Schmidt E. Essential oils, part IV: contact allergy. Dermatitis 2016;27(4):170–5.

28. Corazza M, Borghi A, Gallo R, et al. Topical botanically derived products: use, skin reactions, and usefulness of patch tests. A multicentre Italian study. Contact Dermatitis 2014;70(2):90–7.

29. Gilissen L, Huygens S, Goossens A. Allergic contact dermatitis caused by topical herbal remedies: importance of patch testing with the patients' own products. Contact Dermatitis 2018;78(3):177–84.

30. Paulsen E, Chistensen LP, Andersen KE. Cosmetics and herbal remedies with Compositae plant extracts–are they tolerated by Compositae-allergic patients? Contact Dermatitis 2008;58(1):15–23.

31. Svedman C, Engfeldt M, Api AM, et al. A pilot study aimed at finding a suitable eugenol concentration for a leave-on product for use in a repeated open application test. Contact Dermatitis 2012;66(3):137–9.

32. Fragrances in cosmetics. Available at: https://www.fda.gov/cosmetics/cosmetic-ingredients/fragrances-cosmetics. Accessed July 8, 2019.

33. Perfume allergies. Available at: https://ec.europa.eu/health/scientific_committees/opinions_layman/perfume-allergies/en/l-3/1-introduction.htm. Accessed August 15, 2019.

34. Xu S, Kwa M, Lohman ME, et al. Consumer preferences, product characteristics, and potentially allergenic ingredients in best-selling moisturizers. JAMA Dermatol 2017;153(11):1099–105.

35. Contact allergy management program. Available at: http://www.acdscamp.org/Search_Allergen. Accessed August 8, 2019.

Systemic Contact Dermatitis: A review

Francesca Y. Baruffi, BS[a,1], Kaushik P. Venkatesh, BS[a,1], Kamaria N. Nelson, MD, MHS[b], Alva Powell, BS[a], Diana M. Santos, BS[b], Alison Ehrlich, MD, MHS[c,*]

KEYWORDS

- Patch test • Systemic contact dermatitis • Avoidance diets • Baboon syndrome • Hypersensitivity
- Allergens/immunology • SNAS

KEY POINTS

- The etiology of systemic contact dermatitis (SCD) is most widely considered to be the result of a type IV hypersensitivity reaction and its symptoms are varied.
- The most common culprits associated with SCD include various plants, foods, metals, and medications.
- Patch testing commonly is used to diagnose specific agents causing atopic contact dermatitis; however, it is less useful for SCD due to inferior absorption of some SCD-causing agents into skin.
- Current treatments of SCD include avoidance diets, immunosuppressive agents, phototherapy, and hyposensitization therapy.

INTRODUCTION

Originally termed Baboon syndrome (BS) in 1984, systemic contact dermatitis (SCD) refers to a broad category of syndromes, which share a similar root pathophysiology.[1] At the broadest level, SCD refers to the process by which a patient is first sensitized cutaneously to an allergen and upon reexposure systemically (ie, oral, transcutaneous, subcutaneous, intravenous, intramuscular, rectal, and inhalational) develops a delayed (type IV) hypersensitivity reaction. Along with dermatitis, sequelae as a result of systemic exposure include general malaise, vomiting, diarrhea, arthralgias, and other nonspecific symptoms.[2] Epidemiologic data are difficult to ascertain, because SCD comprises a wide variety of clinical presentations and offending agents.[2] Common allergens can be divided into the following major categories: plants, foods, metals, and drugs; these are discussed in more detail in this review (**Tables 1 and 2**).

DEFINITIONS

There are several categories of SCD, which have been derived from the original Baboon syndrome, which was coined by Andersen and colleagues.[1] The following are the main existing subcategories of SCD:

1. BS
2. Systemic drug-related intertriginous and flexural exanthema (SDRIFE)
3. Allergic contact dermatitis syndrome (ACDS)
4. Systemic nickel allergy syndrome (SNAS)

Many of these terms are used interchangeably and are not well defined or standardized according to any guidelines.

Baboon Syndrome

BS was coined in 1984 by Andersen and colleagues,[1] denoting the clinical picture of a patient who acutely developed a specific pattern of

---

[a] The George Washington School of Medicine and Health Sciences, Washington, DC, USA; [b] Department of Dermatology, The George Washington Medical Faculty Associates, Washington, DC, USA; [c] Foxhall Dermatology, 4910 Massachusetts Avenue NW, Washington, DC 20016, USA
[1] Equal Contributors.
* Corresponding author.
E-mail address: contactderm4dc@gmail.com

Dermatol Clin 38 (2020) 379–388
https://doi.org/10.1016/j.det.2020.02.008
0733-8635/20/

Table 1
Plants and food that induce systemic contact dermatitis

Plants	Common Sources	Foods	Common Sources
Arnica	Homeopathic remedies	Aspartame	Diet beverages, diet candies, and protein powders
Artichoke		Propolis	Cosmetics, syrups, and lozenges
BOP	Citrus fruits, cinnamon, vanilla, cloves, curry, allspice, anise, ketchup, wine, beer, gin, chocolate, colas, and ice cream	Propylene glycol	Drink mixes, creamers, dressings, sauces, baking mixes, fast foods, prepackaged breakfast foods, dried soup mixes, frozen vegetables, ketchup, cereals, and juices
Cashew		Sorbic acid	Beverages, ketchup, salsas, dressings, cereals, baking mixes, toothpaste, prunes, cheeses, and strawberries
Chrysanthemum	Teas	Benzoates	Canned vegetables, sauces, cereals, packaged breads, beverages, butter, cottage cheese, canned and instant soups, and artificial sweeteners
Echinacea	Supplements and teas		
Feverfew	Homeopathic remedies		
Flaxseed			
Garlic			
Mango			
Marigold			
Pistachio			
Poison ivy			
Poison oak			
Ragweed			
Rhus	Chicken coating (Korea)		
Sunflower			
Vanillins			

Data from Refs.[2,7,13,16,20]

erythematous exanthema in the inguinal area, flexural areas, and notably the buttocks area. The erythema usually is well defined and associated with burning and itching and also may present with overlying papules, pustules, and vesicles. Initially Andersen and colleagues[1] specifically reported cases of BS due to heavy metals and drugs, and the list of sensitizing agents has since grown to include foods and plants (see **Table 1**).[1] Miyahara and colleagues[3] more recently divided BS into subcategories based on the agent and mode of sensitization: classical BS; topical drug–induced BS; systemic drug–induced BS, and SDRIFE (discussed later).[3] Other

syndromes that mimic BS but originate from a separate etiology have been described and are termed, infection-induced BS-like pattern and BS-like pattern.

Systemic Drug-related Intertriginous and Flexural Exanthema

Posed by Hauserman and colleagues in 2004,[4] SDRIFE describes a specifically drug-induced reaction, with distinct clinical diagnostic characteristics: (1) first or repeat exposure to a drug via systemic administration; (2) erythema of the inguinal and/or gluteal region; (3) additional

Table 2
Metals that induce systemic contact dermatitis

Metals	Common Sources
Nickel	Beans, lentils, shellfish, chocolate, peanuts, coffee, spinach, soy, drinking water, coins, jewelry, tools, and nickel-plated devices
Cobalt	Flaxseeds, chickpeas, chocolate, nuts, vitamin B_{12}, jewelry, leather, toys, orthopedic devices, and hard metals
Chromium	Potatoes, meats, tea, nuts, grapes, nutritional supplements, multivitamins, dyes, metallurgy, and cement
Zinc	Dental fillings, paint, batteries, and anticorrosive agents
Gold	Jewelry, dental restoration material, and intramuscular injections
Mercury	Seafood and broken thermometers, dental fillings, medications, vaccines, fluorescent lamps, and makeup products
Copper	Dental devices and contraceptive IUDs

Data from Refs.[2,7,13]

erythema of a flexural/intertriginous region; (4) symmetry of areas of erythema; and (5) lack of systemic signs and symptoms. SDRIFE is seen specifically in response to antibiotics, in particular β-lactams and aminopenicillins.[5]

Allergic Contact Dermatitis Syndrome

In 2009, SCD was classified by Özkaya[6] by stages of ACDS. Özkaya proposed that there were 3 stages of ACDS: contact allergenic-induced BS (nondrug); contact allergenic drug-induced BS; and noncontact allergenic drug-induced BS.[6] Contact allergenic-induced BS (nondrug) and contact allergenic drug-induced BS are the result of cutaneously presensitized individuals responding to systemic reexposure. Noncontact allergenic drug-induced BS is analogous to SDRIFE and is classified as a delayed hypersensitivity reaction that does not require previous cutaneous sensitization to elicit a subsequent reaction.[3,6]

Systemic Nickel Allergy Syndrome

SNAS is a subtype of SCD that is characterized by a cutaneous reaction in response to parenteral exposure to nickel in the form of nickel ingestion, implant devices, and inhalation. A type of SCD that is particular to nickel ingestion, SNAS has been suggested to be the result of various immunologic responses to nickel.[7] Jensen and colleagues[8] in 2004 attempted to clarify these responses by conducting a double-blind, placebo-controlled study, which examined nickel-sensitive versus non–nickel-sensitive patients who were exposed orally to varying levels of nickel or placebo. The study found an oral dose–dependent cutaneous response as well as increased levels of postexposure T lymphocytes in nickel-sensitive individuals.[8] Symptoms of SNAS also may include generalized dermatitis, eczema, or an SDRIFE-like cutaneous reaction.[7]

ETIOLOGY

SCD previously has been confused clinically with type I hypersensitivity reactions, but there is a general consensus that SCD and its subcategories are the result of a type IV (and less commonly, type III) hypersensitivity reaction in which a previously sensitized individual undergoes a cytotoxic $CD8^+$ T-cell response upon systemic reexposure.[7] This systemic reexposure encompasses myriad routes, including oral, subcutaneous, intramuscular, inhalation, anal, and other noncutaneous routes of contact. Although incompletely understood, several theories on the pathophysiology of SCD have been proposed. Certain studies suggest that although the basic mechanistic framework remains the same, different cytokines and signaling molecules are paired with specific allergens and that superimposed type I hypersensitivity reactions may concur with SCD, further confusing the clinical picture.[7]

The classical etiology of SCD presents as a type IV hypersensitivity reaction, in which prior cutaneous sensitization results in $CD8^+$ cytotoxic cell migration to the skin after antigen-presenting cells induce a response.[2] Posadas and colleagues[9] most recently proposed the pharmacologic-immune (p-i) theory in 2007 to describe the pathophysiology of SCD to explain drugs that induce a reaction without prior exposure. The sensitizing drug or chemical enters the epidermis as a prohapten, which activates dendritic and Langerhans cells; these cells subsequently migrate to lymph nodes and present as hapten-protein complexes to T cells, which are stimulated and react to induce the cytotoxic response.[9]

SCD is caused by a wide variety of plants and foods, metals, and medications. In the remainder of this article, the top culprits associated with SCD and its subcategories are explored. The most common plants and foods include balsam of Peru (BOP), propolis, chamomile, aspartame, urushiol, propylene glycol, and potassium sorbate. Metals that are known to cause SCD include nickel, chromium, gold, mercury, zinc, and chromium; this category includes SCD caused by metal device implants.[10] Lastly, medications associated most frequently with SCD include various antibiotics and oral and topical steroids.[2]

PLANTS AND FOODS
Balsam of Peru

One of the most commonly known triggers for SCD, BOP, is derived from the sap of the tree species *Myroxylon balsamum pereirae*.[11] It is found in medicine and as a flavoring compound in many foods (see **Table 1**). BOP often is cross-allergenic with vanillins, citrus, cinnamon, garlic, and tomatoes.[12] Certain patients with positive patch testing for fragrance have been shown to have SCD in response to these cross-allergens, specifically cinnamates and vanillins.[13] A case report by Pfützner and colleagues[14] documented 2 patients who were patch-test positive to a mixture of BOP group allergens, including fragrance, who, on oral rechallenge with BOP, developed eczema of the hands, neck, chest, and upper arms.

Propolis

Propolis is a resin compound derived from the sap of various trees and plants and it is related to BOP. It is utilized by bees to construct hives and commonly is referred to as bee glue.[10] Commercially, it is used as an ingredient in oral products, such as toothpaste and lozenges, soaps, lotions, and tinctures for various health remedies.[15] It has been shown via patch testing to be cross-reactive with BOP.[13]

Chamomile

Chamomile is a plant within the Compositae family, which also includes lettuce, artichoke, dandelion, chicory, and tarragon. Compositae species contain sesquiterpene lactones, which are molecules important for plant metabolism. These molecules are strongly binding haptens, which explains their role in the pathogenesis of SCD. Several anecdotal cases of SCD in response to ingestion of Compositae and sunflower species have been reported.[13] Common presentations of SCD in

relation to chamomile and cross-reactive plants include cheilitis, stomatitis, and lip swelling.[16] SCD has been observed in numerous members of the Compositae family, which include lettuce, artichoke, spices, and teas (see **Table 1**).

Aspartame

Aspartame is an artificial sweetener that is metabolized by the liver into a well-known allergic contact dermatitis antigen, formaldehyde.[13] It has been documented in a small number of patients who ingest large quantities of aspartame, such as those found in diet sodas and foods designated as low-fat. The most notable case presentation is an eyelid dermatitis.[17]

Urushiol

Urushiol is a chemical compound found in common foods, such as raw cashews and Rhus sap.[18] These compounds also cross-react with common sources of contact dermatitis, such as poison ivy and poison oak.[13] Rhus chicken, a popular food consisting of roasted chicken covered in a Rhus (urushiol) coating, is commonly ingested in Korea for therapeutic purposes for gastrointestinal issues, and several cases of SCD in response to Rhus chicken have been reported. The most common manifestation of SCD due to ingestion of Rhus chicken is an erythematous maculopapular rash on the trunk and extremities.[13,19]

Propylene Glycol

Commonly known as the major ingredient in antifreeze, propylene glycol is a chemical compound that also is used as a common food additive in processed foods. It is used as a thickening agent and humectant in foods, such as salad dressings, coffee creamers, canned beans, packaged dairy products, cake mixes, and a host of other processed food items[20] (see **Table 1**). Manifestations of propylene-glycol induced SCD include irritation and flaring at previous patch-testing sites as well as eczematous plaques located on the face, hands, and neck.[13]

Sorbic Acid/Potassium Sorbate

Sorbic acid is a natural organic compound that is found in many red fruits, such as strawberries. A synthetic derivative, potassium sorbate, is used as a preservative in foods, such as prunes and cheese.[2,21] Potassium sorbate also is used as a preservative compound in medical and cosmetic products. A case study introduced by Dejobert and colleagues[21] described a patient who presented with a vesicular rash of the hands and feet, who subsequently had a positive patch test to sorbic acid. The patient's rash cleared upon avoidance of foods containing sorbic acid and reappeared upon reintroduction of strawberries, prunes, and margarine.

METALS
Nickel

Nickel is one of the most commonly reported and studied sensitizers that triggers SCD, explained by its ubiquitous presence in the environment and in ingestible foods.[22,23] Nickel sensitization has been reported in up to 17% of women and 3% of men.[10,24] Patient presentations have varied widely but include vesicular hand dermatitis, pruritic papules, generalized dermatitis, and localized dermatitis at a previously sensitized site.[13,25,26] In the literature, the correlation between SCD and nickel has been called SNAS, a systemic response characterized by cutaneous reaction to submucosal nickel exposure through diet, inhalation, or implanted nickel.[7,27]

Nickel exposure primarily occurs through ingestion of nickel-rich foods. Several case reports, case series, cross-sectional studies, and randomized controlled trials have reported overall improvement in SCD symptoms with low-nickel diets.[22] Adherence to dietary restrictions are difficult, however, and complete elimination of dietary nickel is near impossible.[28] Common foods containing nickel include beans, lentils, shellfish, chocolate, peanuts, and coffee.[13] Moreover, sources of drinking water may contain dramatically different amounts of nickel. Furthermore, the average diet contains approximately 300 µg to 600 µg of nickel per day, enough to trigger SCD symptoms in nickel-sensitive patients.[29] SCD also can be induced by exposure to nickel-containing metal objects, such as coins, jewelry, tools, and nickel-plated devices.[2,23]

Cobalt

Cobalt is a metal that frequently is reported to cause SCD. Several studies have found cobalt and nickel cosensitization, with an allergy to one metal increasing sensitivity to the other metal.[30,31] A study by Rystedt and Fischer[32] found that approximately 25% of nickel-sensitized patients also developed cobalt sensitivity. Clinical presentations of cobalt-induced SCD include dyshidrotic eczema flares and generalized eczematous eruptions.[33,34]

Cobalt is present in a variety of foods, including flaxseeds, chickpeas, chocolate, and nuts.[1,2] It also is the main component of vitamin B_{12}, making it clinically relevant to patients on multivitamin supplementation.[35,36] Cobalt also is contained in a plethora of materials, including jewelry, leather, toys, and orthopedic implants.[37] Occupational exposure to cobalt in hard metal manufacturing has been a concerning, although rare cause of SCD. Hard metals often contain cobalt as a binding agent.[23,34,38] Several studies have found that dietary avoidance results in overall improvement of dermatitis.[39–41]

Chromium

Chromium and chromate are the cause of approximately 2% of ACD cases.[13] Chromium is an essential trace element found in water, air, and soil. Skin contact with hexavalent and trivalent chromium compounds as well as ingestion of the dichromate form have been reported to trigger SCD.[42–44] Patient presentations include chronic, recurrent, vesicular hand eczema, and subacute eczematous dermatitis in the lower legs, ankles, and hands.[13,29,33]

Its ubiquity in the biosphere results in a concerning presence in foodstuffs. Chromium is particularly high in potatoes, meats, tea, and nuts.[29] It also commonly is found in nutritional supplements and multivitamins and commonly is used in dye production, metallurgy, and cement.[6,45] Chromium avoidance diets have been documented to improve dermatitis in several studies.[39–41,46]

Zinc

Zinc is an essential trace element with several biological functions and is widely used in dental work and industrial applications (paint, batteries, and anticorrosive agents).[10] Zinc may be absorbed both through dietary intake and through the skin or oral mucosa.[23] Dietary zinc sources include almonds, chocolates, cheeses, liver, and oysters.[47] Documented clinical presentations include generalized vesicular rashes, pruritic skin eruptions, and oral lichen planus.[48–50]

A few studies and case reports have reported that zinc avoidance diets are successful in controlling SCD symptoms.[39,47] Other investigators have reported the removal of the allergen from dental fillings have improved flares associated with the dental work procedures.[41]

Gold

Gold has several uses, including its composition in jewelry, density restoration material, and intramuscular injections in anti-inflammatory therapy for rheumatoid arthritis.[10,51] It also can be found in some foods and beverages.[10] Although relatively rare, several cases of gold-induced SCD have been reported, such as SCD induced by homeopathic drug Aurocard after previous sensitization to gold earrings and a dental crown, rheumatoid arthritis treatment injections, and several others.[51-56] Gold sometimes may present as late reactions in patch testing and can be especially challenging to diagnose if late readings are not performed 7 or more days later. It is recommended to follow-up with patients for up to 3 weeks after patch testing to evaluate late reactions.[51,54,57]

Mercury

Mercury is the earliest metal discovered to cause SCD.[1] SCD was thought to be triggered by systemic absorption of mercury vapors from thermometers or ingestion of mercury in dental fillings or medications.[3,58] Previous sensitization usually would occur from other mercury compounds, for example, mercurochrome, ophthalmic preparations, disinfectant medications, and vaccines.[3,10,59-61] Fortunately, mercury use has declined in recent years given toxicity concerns, although it still is present in the production of chlorine and caustic soda, some thermometers, fluorescent lamps, makeup products (mascara), and certain high-mercury foods (seafood).[10]

Common clinical presentations include the typical BS phenotype, with primary presentation in the flexural areas.[3] Mercury-related SCD has been reported more frequently in some Western European countries and Southeast Asian countries.[3] This may be due, however, to the persistence of usage of mercury in instruments, such as thermometers.[3]

Copper

Copper rarely is reported as an allergen for SCD. It commonly is used in dental devices and contraceptive intrauterine devices (IUDs). Evidence of delayed-type stomatitis has been reported from copper in dental devices.[51] Copper in IUDs also has induced SCD in copper-sensitive women.[62,63]

Biomedical Devices

Erosion and corrosion of metal implants release free ions proximal to the implant and systemically. Numerous types of metal implants have been implicated in SCD, including orthopedic implants, endovascular devices, pacemakers, Nuss pectus implant, dental implants, and IUDs. These devices consist of a variety of potential allergenic materials, including stainless steel (chromium, molybdenum, and nickel), titanium (vanadium and aluminum), nitinol (nickel), chromium/cobalt alloy, dental amalgam (mercury, gold, and nickel), and IUD copper sulfate.[64] The literature reports nickel as the greatest concern among biomedical devices, with nitinol releasing the least free nickel and stainless steel releasing the most.[65] Several studies suggest that patch testing should be considered preimplantation in high risk patients to screen for potential sensitivities.[65-67]

MEDICATIONS

Medications are another leading cause of SCD and include a variety of topical and systemic medications.[10] When medications lead to SCD, skin lesions are characterized by an erythematous morbilliform eruption involving the buttocks and flexural areas in a symmetric distribution.[2,35] This skin eruption is of similar presentation to SDRIFE. SCD should be distinguished from other drug-induced skin eruptions, including fixed drug eruption, drug reaction with eosinophilia and systemic symptoms, and acute generalized exanthematous pustulosis (AGEP).

There have been numerous drugs associated with the development of SCD, with the most common being antibiotics, such as amoxicillin, ceftriaxone, penicillin, clindamycin, and erythromycin. Topical and oral corticosteroids also are a common cause of SCD and reactions to systemic corticosteroids can occur even without prior cutaneous exposure.[2] Furthermore, there have been case reports of steroids causing a more bullous eruption as opposed to a morbilliform eruption.[68] Other medications include anesthetics, antihistamine, aminophylline, 5-aminosalicylic acid, and bufexamac.[10] Gold has previously been used in some medications for treatment of rheumatoid arthritis and can be found in homeopathic remedies and shown to cause SCD.[2,52]

DIAGNOSIS

SCD has a wide variety of differential diagnoses. In pediatric patients, it is important to rule out viral exanthems, impetigo, perianal cellulitis, and staphylococcal scalded skin syndrome. Other differentials with similar localization include Hailey-Hailey disease, pemphigus vegetans (localized form of pemphigus vulgaris), inverse psoriasis, candidiasis, tinea cruris, AGEP, SDRIFE, irritant contact dermatitis, and allergic contact dermatitis.[10] Use of clinical presentation, patient history, and specific allergy tests can help differentiate between the various diagnoses.[2,10]

Patch Testing

Epicutaneous patch testing has been relatively successful in identifying allergens causing both ACD and SCD reactions to materials such as metal, medications, and plant hypersensitivities.

It can be performed with either a standard series panel or a customized panel with the allergens of interest. The adaptability of patch testing allows various potential allergens to be tested. Some medications, for example, certain corticosteroids, antimicrobials, nonsteroidal anti-inflammatory drugs, anesthetics, and antihistamines, already are commercially produced for patch.[2] For drugs without commercially prepared allergens available for patch testing, the European Society of Contact Dermatitis has created detailed and applicable guidelines for patch testing of medications.[69] Metals, plants, herbals, and other various allergens also can be patch tested effectively.[70] For metal biomedical devices, Schalock and colleagues[67] suggest using a metal series depending on the implant type and patient history.

Although patch testing is the gold standard for ACD, SCD may present challenges due to inferior absorption of systemically administered drugs through the skin. Additionally, accuracy of this test is limited by evaluator experience, and differentiating false-positive and true-positive reactions remains difficult for various allergens. Moreover, some metal salts have resulted in irritant reactions and false-positives.[71] SDRIFE-causing compounds, such as antibiotics (aminopenicillins and β-lactams) often are patch test negative in up to half of cases.[4,5] This may be an advantage because patch testing can allow clinicians to differentiate between SCD and other drug-induced eruptions without previous sensitization, such as SDRIFE.[10]

TREATMENT

Treatment of SCD involves allergen avoidance as determined by clinical history and patch testing results. Skin findings usually resolve within a few weeks after avoidance of culprit allergens. Topical corticosteroids may be useful for mild skin inflammation and pruritus, and oral corticosteroids may be used for more severe cases.[10]

Avoidance diets are considered in combination with oral food challenges to determine if allergic symptoms resolve once the suspected allergens are removed from the diet. The avoidance diet can be created based on clinical history and serves as a diagnostic adjunct.[72] Patients who have SCD toward nickel and whose symptoms do not resolve with contact avoidance should consider a low nickel diet and should avoid foods high in nickel, such as shellfish, seafood, chocolate, legumes, grains, and nuts. When possible, patients should avoid canned foods and nickel-containing cookware. Patients with SCD to BOP should avoid fragrances and may show improvement with avoiding foods that contain BOP, such as citrus fruits, cinnamon, ketchup, pickles, wine, beer, gin, chocolate, ice cream, tomatoes, and spiced soft drinks. Some patients may benefit from a low chromate diet if they have SCD to chromium. Recommendations include abstaining from items, such as whole grains, potatoes, foods packaged in aluminum products, meats with high concentrations of chromium, and hard tap water. Fresh fruits and tea/coffee should be consumed in moderation. Avoidance diets for cobalt, propylene glycol, and aspartame allergies also have been described.[2]

For recalcitrant cases, immunosuppressive agents may be used to manage SCD in patients who fail topical corticosteroids or avoidance diets. These agents include azathioprine, cyclosporine, methotrexate, and mycophenolate mofetil.[12] Disulfiram, a nickel and cobalt chelator, more commonly used for alcohol dependence, has been used with varying success for nickel systemic contact allergy.[12,73] Phototherapy is another option for difficult cases and includes narrowband UV-B, UV-A, and topical or systemic psoralen with UV-A. Phototherapy should be avoided in patients with UV sensitivity or with a personal history of malignant melanoma.[12] Hyposensitization is an emerging therapy for SCD that involves increasing amounts of allergen exposure in an attempt to alter the immune response. In nickel oral hyposensitization, it is thought that upon increasing exposure there are changes to the T-cell regulatory response leading to an increase in interleukin 10 and increased tolerance to the allergen.[12,74,75] Patients undergoing hyposensitization should be monitored closely for adverse events.

SUMMARY

SCD is relatively rare and is characterized by cutaneous eruption in response to systemic allergen exposure after previous cutaneous sensitization. Systemic exposure can occur via a variety of routes, from dietary intake to prosthetic implants. Its mechanism is not fully understood, although evidence suggests that it is mediated via type IV hypersensitivity reaction. The p-i concept also recently has been proposed to explain SCD's unique first-exposure and delayed-type reactions. Diagnosis remains difficult with SCD's diversity of presentations. Epicutaneous patch testing remains the gold standard for diagnosis, though observer experience is important for proper interpretation. Oral challenges and avoidance diets also may prove useful in eliciting allergen dosing and reactivity information. Flares remain a major concern during diagnosis due to reexposure to the allergen. Treatments include allergy avoidance and corticosteroids, when indicated. For cases refractory to corticosteroids, treatment may utilize artificial UV phototherapy or systemic immunosuppressants, such as cyclosporine, azathioprine, and methotrexate.[76] Overall, future studies are needed to better understand the pathophysiology, potential allergens, diagnosis, and avoidance diet treatments of SCD.

DISCLOSURE

The authors have nothing to disclose.

REFERENCES

1. Andersen KE, Hjorth N, Menne T. The baboon syndrome: systemically-induced allergic contact dermatitis. Contact Dermatitis 1984;10:97–100.
2. Aquino M, Rosner G. Systemic contact dermatitis. Clin Rev Allergy Immunol 2019;56(1):9–18.
3. Miyahara A, Kawashima H, Okubo Y, et al. A new proposal for a clinical-oriented subclassification of baboon syndrome and a review of baboon syndrome. Asian Pac J Allergy Immunol 2011;29: 150–60.
4. Hauserman P, Harr T, Bircher AJ. Baboon syndrome resulting from systemic drugs: is there strife between SDRIFE and allergic contact dermatitis syndrome? Contact Dermatitis 2004;51(5–6):297–310.
5. Winnicki M, Shear N. A systematic approach to systemic contact dermatitis and symmetric drug-related intertriginous and flexural exanthema (SDRIFE): a closer look at these conditions and an approach to intertriginous eruptions. Am J Clin Dermatol 2011;12(3):171–80.
6. Özkaya E. Current understanding of baboon syndrome. Expert Rev Dermatol 2009;4(2):163–75.
7. Rundle CW, Machler BC, Jacob SE. Pathogenesis and causations of systemic contact dermatitis. G Ital Dermatol Venereol 2019;154(1):42–9.
8. Jensen CS, Lisby S, Larsen JK, et al. Characterization of lymphocyte subpopulations and cytokine profiles in peripheral blood of nickel-sensitive individuals with systemic contact dermatitis after oral nickel exposure. Contact Dermatitis 2004; 50(1):31–8.
9. Posadas S, Pichler W. Delayed drug hypersensitivity reactions new concepts. Clin Exp Allergy 2007; 37(7):989–99.
10. Kulberg A, Schliemann S, Elsner P. Contact dermatitis as a systemic disease. Clin Dermatol 2014;32: 414–9.
11. Katta R, Schlichte M. Diet and dermatitis: Food triggers. J Clin Aesthet Dermatol 2014;7(3):30–6.

12. Lampel H, Silvestri D. Systemic contact dermatitis: current challenges and emerging treatments. Curr Treat Options Allergy 2014;1(4):348–57.
13. Fabbro S, Zirwas M. Systemic contact dermatitis to foods: nickel, bop, and more. Curr Allergy Asthma Rep 2014;14(10):463.
14. Pfützner W, Thomas P, Niedermeier A, et al. Systemic contact dermatitis elicited by oral intake of Balsam of Peru. Acta Derm Venereol 2003;83(4): 294–5.
15. Cho E, Lee JD, Cho SH. Systemic contact dermatitis from propolis ingestion. Ann Dermatol 2011;23(1): 85–8.
16. Paulsen E. Systemic allergic dermatitis caused by sesquiterpene lactones. Contact Dermatitis 2017; 76(1):1–10.
17. Hill AM, Belsito DV. Systemic contact dermatitis of the eyelids caused by formaldehyde derived from aspartame? Contact Dermatitis 2003;49(5): 258–9.
18. Cheong SH, Choi YW, Min BS, et al. Polymerized urushiol of the commercially available Rhus product in Korea. Ann Dermatol 2010;22(1):16–20.
19. Yoo KH, Seo SJ, Li K, et al. Ingestion of Rhus chicken causing systemic contact dermatitis in a Korean patient. Clin Exp Dermatol 2010;35(7): 756–8.
20. Scheman A, Cha C, Jacob SE, et al. Food avoidance diets for systemic, lip, and oral contact allergy: an American contact alternatives group article. Dermatitis 2012;23(6):248–57.
21. Dejobert Y, Delaporte E, Piette F, et al. Vesicular eczema and systemic contact dermatitis from sorbic acid. Contact Dermatitis 2001;45(5):291.
22. Scott J, Hammond M, Nedorost S. Food avoidance diets for dermatitis. Curr Allergy Asthma Rep 2015; 15(10):1–13.
23. Yoshihisa Y, Shimizu T. Metal allergy and systemic contact dermatitis: an overview. Dermatol Res Pract 2012;2012(2012):749561.
24. Benamran S, Votadoro A, Sleth JC. Acute systemic contact dermatitis in a patient with nickel hypersensitivity: contamination from an intravenous catheter? Acta Anaesthesiol Scand 2007;51:647–8.
25. Lu LK, Warshaw EM, Dunnick CA. Prevention of nickel allergy: the case for regulation? Dermatol Clin 2009;27(2):155–61.
26. Veien NK. Ingested food in systemic allergic contact dermatitis. Clin Dermatol 1997;15(4):547–55.
27. Da Mata Perez L, França AT, Zimmerman JR. Systemic nickel allergy syndrome. World Allergy Organ J 2015;8(Suppl 1):A89.
28. Antico A, Soana R. Nickel sensitization and dietary nickel are a substantial cause of symptoms provocation in patients with chronic allergic-like dermatitis syndromes. Allergy Rhinol (Providence) 2015;6(1): 56–63.

29. Sharma AD. Low nickel diet in dermatology. Indian J Dermatol 2013;58:240.

30. Veien NK, Hattel T, Justesen O, et al. Oral challenge with nickel and cobalt in patients with positive patch tests to nickel and/or cobalt. Acta Derm Venereol 1987;67(4):321–5.

31. Veien NK, Hattel T, Laurberg G. Placebo-controlled oral challenge with cobalt in patients with positive patch tests to cobalt. Contact Dermatitis 1995; 33(1):54–5.

32. Rystedt I, Fischer T. Relationship between nick and cobalt sensitization in hard metal workers. Contact Dermatitis 1983;9(3):195–200.

33. Stuckert J, Nedorost S. Low-cobalt diet for dyshidrotic eczema patients. Contact Dermatitis 2008; 59(6):361–5.

34. Asano Y, Makino T, Norisugi O, et al. Occupational cobalt induced systemic contact dermatitis. Eur J Dermatol 2009;19(2):166–8.

35. Jacob SE, Zapolanski T. Systemic contact dermatitis. Dermatitis 2008;19(1):9–15.

36. Fisher AA. Contact dermatitis at home and abroad. Cutis 1972;10:719.

37. Fowler JF. Cobalt. Dermatitis 2016;27(1):3–8.

38. Schwartz L, Peck SM, Blair KE, et al. Allergic dermatitis due to metallic cobalt. J Allergy 1945;16(1):51–3.

39. Adachi A, Horikawa T, Takashima T, et al. Potential efficacy of low metal diets and dental metal elimination in the management of atopic dermatitis: an open clinical study. J Dermatol 1997;24(1):12–9.

40. Veien NK, Hattel T, Justesen O, et al. Oral challenge with metal salts. (I). Vesicular patch-test-negative hand eczema. Contact Dermatitis 1983;9(5):402–6.

41. Veien NK, Hattel T, Justesen O, et al. Oral challenge with metal salts. (II). Various types of eczema. Contact Dermatitis 1983;9(5):407–10.

42. Hansen MB, Johansen JD, Menné T. Chromium allergy: significance of both Cr(III) and Cr(VI). Contact Dermatitis 2003;49(4):206–12.

43. Kaaber K, Veien NK. The significance of chromate ingestion in patients allergic to chromate. Acta Derm Venereol 1977;57(4):321–3.

44. Veien NK, Hattel R, Laurberg G. Chromate allergic patients challenged orally with potassium dichromate. Contact Dermatitis 1994;31(3):137–9.

45. Burrows D. Adverse chromate reactions on the skin. In: Burrows D, editor. Chromium: metabolism and toxicity. Boca Raton (FL): CRC Press; 2000. p. 137–63.

46. Sharma A. Low chromate diet in dermatology. Indian J Dermatol 2009;54(3):293–5.

47. Sakai T, Hatano Y, Fujiwara S. Systemic contact dermatitis due to zinc successfully treated with a zinc-restricted diet: a case report. Allergol Int 2013;62(2):265–7.

48. Shimizu T, Kobayashi S, Tanaka M. Systemic contact dermatitis to zinc in dental fillings. Clin Exp Dermatol 2003;28(676):675.

49. Saito N, Yamane N, Matsumura W, et al. Generalized exacerbation of systemic allergic dermatitis due to zinc patch test and dental treatments. Contact Dermatitis 2010;62(6):372–3.

50. Ido T, Kumakiri M, Kiyohara T, et al. Oral lichen planus due to zinc in dental restorations. Contact Dermatitis 2002;47(1):51.

51. Hostynek JJ. Gold: an allergen of growing significance. Food Chem Toxicol 1997;35(8):839–44.

52. Malinauskiene I, Isaksson M, Bruze M. Systemic contact dermatitis in a gold-allergic patient after treatment with an oral homeopathic drug. J Am Acad Dermatol 2013;68:e58.

53. Wicks IP, Wong D, McCullagh RB, et al. Contact allergy to gold after systemic administration of gold for rheumatoid arthritis. Ann Rheum Dis 1998;47(5):421–2.

54. Moller H. Contact allergy to gold as a model for clinical-experimental research. Contact Dermatitis 2010;62:193–200.

55. Moller H, Ohlsson K, Linder C, et al. Cytokines and acute phase reactants during flare-up of contact allergy to gold. Am J Contact Dermat 1998;9:15–22.

56. Moller H, Ohlsson K, Linder C, et al. The flare-up reactions after systemic provocation in contact allergy to nickel and gold. Contact Dermatitis 1999;40:200–4.

57. Nijhawan R, Molenda M, Zirwas M, et al. Systemic contact dermatitis. Dermatol Clin 2009;27(3):355–64.

58. Veien NK. Stomatitis and systemic dermatitis from mercury in amalgam dental restorations. Dermatol Clin 1990;8(1):157–60.

59. Barrazza V, Meunier P, Escande JP. Acute contact dermatitis and exanthematous pustulosis due to mercury. Contact Dermatitis 1998;38:361.

60. Vena GA, Foti C, Grandolfo M, et al. Mercury exanthema. Contact Dermatitis 1994;31:214–6.

61. Lerch M, Bircher AJ. Systemically induced allergic exanthema from mercury. Contact Dermatitis 2004; 50:349–53.

62. Barranco VP. Eczematous dermatitis caused by internal exposure to copper. Arch Dermatol 1972; 106(3):386–7.

63. Zabel M, Lindscheid KR, Mark H. Copper sulfate allergy with special reference to internal exposure. Z Hautkr 1990;65(5):481–6.

64. Aquino M, Mucci T. Systemic contact dermatitis and allergy to biomedical devices. Curr Allergy Asthma Rep 2013;13(5):518–27.

65. Honari G, Ellis SG, Wilkoff BL, et al. Hypersensitivity reactions associated with endovascular devices. Contact Dermatitis 2008;59(1):7–22.

66. Reed KB, Davis MD, Nakamura K, et al. Retrospective evaluation of patch testing before or after metal device implantation. Arch Dermatol 2008;144(8):999–1007.

67. Schalock PC, Menne T, Johansen JD, et al. Hypersensitivity reactions to metallic implants - diagnostic

algorithm and suggested patch test series for clinical use. Contact Dermatitis 2012;66(1):4–19.

68. Gumaste PV, Cohen DE, Stein JA. Bullous systemic contact dermatitis caused by an intra-articular steroid injection. Br J Dermatol 2015;172(1):300–2.

69. Barbaud A, Goncalo M, Bruynzeel D, et al. Guidelines for performing skin tests with drugs in the investigation of cutaneous adverse drug reactions. Contact Dermatitis 2001;45(6):321–8.

70. Fonacier L, Noor I. Contact dermatitis and patch testing for the allergist. Ann Allergy Asthma Immunol 2018;120(6):592–8.

71. Fischer T, Rystedt I. False-positive, follicular and irritant patch test reactions to metal salts. Contact dermatitis 1985;12(2):93–8.

72. Wood RA. Diagnostic elimination diets and oral food provocation. Chem Immunol Allergy 2015;101: 87–95.

73. Tammaro A, Narcisi A, Persechino S, et al. Topical and systemic therapies for nickel allergy. Dermatitis 2011;22(5):251–5.

74. Ricciardi L, Carni A, Loschiavo G, et al. Systemic nickel allergy: oral desensitization and possible role of cytokines Interleukin 2 and 10. Int J Immunopathol Pharmacol 2013;26(1):251–7.

75. Soyer OU, Akdis M, Akdis CA. Mechanism of subcutaneous allergen immunotherapy. Immunol Allergy Clin N Am 2011;31(2):175–90.

76. Megna M, Napolitano M, Patruno C, et al. Systemic treatment of adult atopic dermatitis: a review. Dermatol Ther 2017;7(1):1–23.

Plant Associated Irritant & Allergic Contact Dermatitis (Phytodermatitis)

Michael P. Sheehan, MD[a,b,*]

KEYWORDS

- Plant • Irritant dermatitis • Allergic dermatitis • Contact dermatitis • Phytodermatitis
- Phytophotodermatitis

KEY POINTS

- Phytodermatitis is skin inflammation induced by contact with plant-derived substances.
- Irritant phytodermatitis is more common than allergic phytodermatitis.
- Phytophotodermatitis is a phototoxic reaction.

INTRODUCTION

Currently there are more than 350,000 plant species recognized and new species are continuing to be identified.[1] Not surprisingly, humans contact plants or plant-containing substances daily. The number of potential botanic exposures is nearly endless. The enormous array of substances and exposures also makes the study of plant dermatitis, also known as phytodermatitis, quite challenging. For example, we may start our day with plant-derived products, such as coffee or tea. Bathing continues the potential for exposures, as many soaps and shampoos sold today contain botanic-derived ingredients. Moisturizers similarly follow the "natural" trend, and may contain substances such as shea butter, which is a fatty substance obtained from the nuts of the shea tree. Other botanicals frequently found in moisturizers include *Aloe vera, Anthemis nobilis, Apis mellifera, Arnica montana, Chamomilla officinalis, Echinacea angustifolia, Echinacea purpurea, Lavandula angustifolia, Matricaria chamomilla*, and ylang-ylang oil derived from *Cananga odorata*,[2] and to this point we have only had a cup of coffee or tea and a shower. With that being said, most isolated and classified plant species are harmless to the skin. What we are concerned with is the smaller group, which may cause irritant (ICD) or allergic contact dermatitis (ACD). It is also important to point out that the risk of developing phytodermatitis depends on the local botanic flora, climate, occupation and life style, and the immune reactivity of the patient.[3] For example, horticulturists, agriculturists, forest and nursery workers, wood workers, cooks, and those who work in the perfume industries are at an increased risk for plant dermatitis.

IRRITANT CONTACT DERMATITIS

As with other forms of contact dermatitis, ICD is more common than ACD from plants. What is somewhat unique is that many plants have a complex structure that affords the ability to induce skin injury through irritant means via several mechanisms. These mechanisms broadly can be considered in 3 main categories: mechanical injury, chemical injury, and phototoxic injury[4] (**Table 1**). Mechanical injury is simply traumatic injury such as may occur from a thorn or splinter. Chemical injury can result from skin exposure to plant substances that are acidic or have enzymatic properties. Bromelain, for example, is a complex mixture of enzymes that was originally isolated form pineapples and found to be a skin irritant. Now it is

[a] Dermatology Physicians, Inc., 360 Plaza Drive, Suite C, Columbus, IN 47201, USA; [b] Department of Dermatology, Indiana University School of Medicine, Indianapolis, IN, USA
* 1725 Washington Street, Columbus, IN 47201, USA.
E-mail address: mpsheeha@iupui.edu

Dermatol Clin 38 (2020) 389–398
https://doi.org/10.1016/j.det.2020.02.010

Table 1
Plant-derived irritants

Substance	Other	Mechanism	Clinical Presentation	Examples
Trichomes and glochids	Also called hairs, barbs, spines, thorns.	Mechanical (traumatic) skin injury.	Papular dermatitis, foreign body granulomas, urticarial dermatitis, pruriginous dermatitis, secondary infection	Agave, blackberry, brambles, cacti, dogwood, forget-me-not, holly, roses, saw palmetto, stinging nettle, thistles, tulip
Alkaloids	Capsaicin, cholchicine, ephedrin, morphine, nicotine, quinolones are all alkaloids.	Various forms of bioactivity (chemical injury).	Daffodil itch	Narcissus (daffodil)
Bromelain	Originally extracted from the pineapple.	Collection of enzymes, including proteases, phosphatases, and peroxidases (chemical injury).	Pineapple worker hand dermatitis	Pineapple
Calcium oxalate	Found in members of more than 215 plant families and may be found in any part of the plant.	Forms bundles of needlelike crystals called raphides that penetrate the skin and enhance penetration of other irritants (mechanical injury).	Irritant bulb sorter dermatitis	Found in numerous ornamental bulbs such as Narcissus (daffodil) and hyacinth; also found in dieffenbachia.
Capsaicin	Type of alkaloid.	Binds vanilloid receptors on sensory neurons (chemical injury).	Hunan hand syndrome, chili burns	Chili peppers
Diterpene esters	Phorbol, daphnane, and diterpene are all diterpene esters and are some of the most irritating plant substances.	Corrosive plant-derived chemicals (chemical injury).	Pain, erythema, edema, and blistering; may cause blindness with ocular contact and severe esophageal trauma with bloody diarrhea with ingestion	Spurges (Euphorbiaceae): poinsettias, manchineel (beach) tree, castor bean plant (*Ricinus communis*)

Juglone	Aromatic naphthoquinone found in the leaves, roots and bark of member of the Juglandaceae family.	Mildly irritating and staining (chemical injury).	Cause of irritant contact dermatitis and noninflammatory hyperpigmentation	Walnut trees
Protoanemonin	Bruising of plant tissue results in ranunculin (a glycoside) being hydrolyzed into protoanemonin.	Volatile unsaturated lactone, which disrupts disulfide bonds in the skin (chemical injury).		Ranunculaceae (buttercup) family
Ricin	Poisonous substance found in the seed but not the oil.	Protein that can cause type I hypersensitivity reactions (chemical injury).	Skin irritation, urticaria, dermatitis, and asthma among castor oil extractors and farmers	Castor bean
Furocoumarin	Psoralen	Phototoxic injury	Erythematous or bullous reactions, hyperpigmentation	Carrot, parsnip, dill, fennel, celery, fig, lime, mokihana

commonly used in the culinary arts as a meat tenderizer. The third category, phytophotodermatitis, is a unique type of ICD induced by phototoxic chemicals contained within plants combined with UV exposure. Plant-derived psoralens (a type of furocoumarin) are typically the cause of phytophotodermatitis.[5] The classic clinical presentation is a patient presenting in the summer or after vacation with linear hyperpigmented patches on exposed skin. Often there is a history of prior painful, red, and often blistered inflammation. On vacation, the source of psoralen exposure is often a lime in a drink, such as margaritas, tequila, or beer. The cutaneous manifestations may occur on perioral skin from consumption or on the hands or arms from inadvertent spilling. Interestingly, pruritus is often not as pronounced as with ACD, which can be helpful in differentiating phytophotodermatitis from other forms of phytodermatitis, such as poison ivy.[5] Other forms of phytophotodermatitis include strimmer dermatitis or weed-eater dermatitis, which results from exposure to psoralens being flung on exposed skin during lawn trimming or weeding.[6] Hawaiian leis containing *Pelea anisate* (Rutaceae family) have also been reported to cause phytophotodermatitis on the neck.[7]

Certain plants are particularly toxic due to their irritant nature. For example, *Dieffenbachia sequine* (**Fig. 1**) is a popular indoor plant that contains a high concentration of the irritant calcium oxalate. The calcium oxalate crystals are water insoluble and are ejected from the plant when exposed to water. If ingested, a severe corrosive glossitis may result.[8] This has resulted in many referring to this plant as "dumb cane," because ingestion will result in losing the ability to talk for several days.

ALLERGIC CONTACT DERMATITIS

Type IV delayed hypersensitivity reactions account for most of plant-induced ACD cases. The responsible haptens are characteristically water insoluble and found within plant resins. Interestingly, the pollen component of plants more often contains water-soluble antigens that play a role in asthma and hay fever but less often in ACD.[9,10] Plant resin is typically referred to as *oleoresin* and may contain more than 500 different chemicals. Aromatic alcohols, aldehydes, and terpenes are some of the more commonly found oleoresin components.[11]

Anacardiaceae

The Anacardiaceae plant family contains the *Toxicodendron* genus. Poison ivy (*Tanacetum radicans, Tanacetum rydbergii*), poison oak (*Tanacetum diversilobum, Tanacetum toxicarium*), and poison sumac (*Tanacetum vernix*) are *Toxicodendron* members. It has been estimated that approximately 50% to 60% of Americans are allergic to poison ivy.[3,12] The leaves of poison ivy and poison oak are trifoliolate, leading to the adage "leaves of three, let them be." Poison sumac has 7 to 13 leaflets. The allergen in the plant oleoresin is a mixture of pentadecylcatechols collectively known as urushiol (**Table 2**). ACD resulting from contact with a member of the *Toxicodendron* genus usually results in the appearance of linear streaks of papulovesicular dermatitis on exposed skin (**Fig. 2**). There may be an initial urticarial phase or a cellulitic appearance. The term "black dot poison ivy" has been applied to forms of more severe ACD in which the black dots or streaks represent dried urushiol on the skin.

Other members of the Anacardiaceae plant family may cross-react with *Toxicodendron* species, including cashew (*Anacardium occidentale*), Indian marking nut (*Semecarpus anacardium*), Japanese lacquer tree (*Rhus vernicifera*), and mango (*Mangifera indica*).[13]

The cashew nut tree (*Anacardium occidentale*) is a small tropical tree that produces the cashew nut as its fruit. The edible portion of the cashew nut is found within its shell and it may be eaten raw or roasted. The shell contains a brown, oily juice

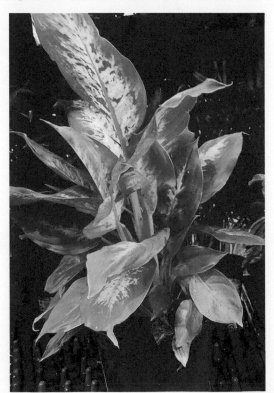

Fig. 1. *Dieffenbachia sequine.*

Table 2
Plant haptens and clinical presentations

Plant	Hapten	Clinical Presentation
Anacardiaceae	Urushiol	Linear streaks of papulovesicular dermatitis on exposed skin; "black dot poison ivy"
Tulip	α-Methylene-γ-butyrolactone (tulipalin A)	Tulip fingers
Narcissus (daffodil)	Unknown	Daffodil itch
Hyacinth	Possibly phenylacetaldehyde (hyacinthine)	Hyacinth itch
Garlic, onion, chive	Allicin and diallyl disulfide	Hyperkeratosis and fissuring of the first 3 fingers on the nondominant hand
Alstroemeria	α-Methylene-γ-butyrolactone (tulipalin A)	Hyperkeratosis and fissuring of the finger tips similar to tulip fingers; depigmentation
Chrysanthemum	Sesquiterpene lactones	Airborne dermatitis, chronic actinic dermatitis
Primrose	Primin (2-methoxy-6-pentylbenzoquinone)	Primula dermatitis
Dalbergia nigra (also known as Brazilian rosewood or jacaranda)	R-4-methoxydalbergione	Dermatitis among woodworkers
Pinaceae	Colophony (also called rosin)	Wide array of presentations and exposures including pine trees, personal care products, topical medicaments, and adhesives
Essential oils derived from evergreen trees	Ylang-ylang, sandalwood	Wide array of presentations and exposures, including trees, personal care products, fragrances, and flavorings
Myroxylon pereirae	*Myroxylon pereirae* (balsam of Peru)	Wide array of presentations and exposures, including trees, personal care products, fragrances, and flavorings

that blackens in the air and is strongly irritating to the skin and may also cause ACD.[3] If the nuts are roasted while in the shell, the fumes can be very irritating to the lungs. A case of systemic ACD has been reported from inhalation of cashew oil smoke after at-home roasting of raw cashew nuts.[14] Occupational desensitization to poison ivy has been reported in cashew nut industry workers[15] as well as paronychia.[16] Unlike many other nuts, most cashews sold to consumers have the shell removed.

The Indian marking nut tree (*S anacardium*) is a moderate-sized deciduous tree native to India that is known for producing the "elephant flea" nut. The black oil (bhilawanol) of this nut is water insoluble and has been used as an ink to label clothing before washing. It has also been used as a varnish.[3] This oil contains a pentadecylcatechol related to poison ivy.[17] In India those who work in textile washing were historically referred to as dhobies and "dhobie mark dermatitis" is seen in persons preparing bhilawanol ink and laundry workers who mark clothing.

The Japanese lacquer tree (*Rhus verniciflua*) is a large tree native to Japan and China. It is cultivated for its dense sap that is used as a urushi lacquer. The art of Japanese lacquerware uses urushi lacquer. This should not be confused with the

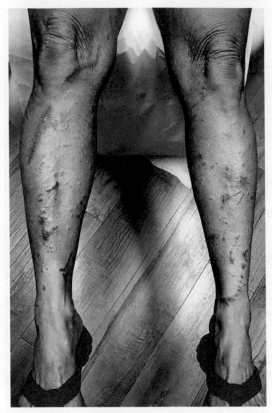

Fig. 2. Poison ivy ACD.

European form of lacquerware called Japanning, which uses a different form of lacquer.

The mango tree (*M indica*) is a large tropical tree cultivated for its fruit, the mango. The mango tree has been used in traditional medicine. Its seeds have antihelminth properties, the brown juice obtained from tree bark has been used to treat diarrhea, and the young leaves have been used for chronic cough and asthma.[3] Urushiol is found in the plant leaves, stems, timber and the fruit pericarp. Collectively, the urushiol components in the mango have been termed "mangol" (heptadecadienylresorcinol, heptadecenylresorcinol, petadecylresorcinol).[18] Mango wood may be used in turning bowls and pens as well as some fine furniture, placing woodworkers at risk. Cheilitis, facial dermatitis, or systemic contact dermatitis may result after ingestion and it has generally been reported that the peel rather than the juice and pulp of the mango were responsible,[19] although others have shown reactions on patch testing to mango pulp.[20]

Bulbous Plants

Ornamental flowers are often implicated in ACD. The tulip is one such ornamental plant, which belongs to the genus *Tulipa* and the family Liliaceae. Tulips bloom each year in the spring and grow from a bulb. Successful growth and cultivation each year requires manual handling, including digging and inspecting the bulbs. Contact dermatitis may result from handling either the bulb or the flower components of the plant. The hapten responsible for eliciting ACD is felt to be α-methylene-γ-butyrolactone, which is found within the glucoside extract tulipalin A.[21–23] The tulip bulb has a rough dry exterior and handling may result in ICD. However, tulip bulbs do not contain appreciable amounts of calcium oxalate crystals, which are felt to be the principal cause of other forms of irritant bulb dermatitis. Occupational exposure from handling tulip bulbs can cause what has been termed "tulip fingers."[24] Patients may report dysesthesias, such as tingling and burning or tenderness, and examination shows pulpitis with hyperkeratosis and fissuring of the fingertips. The thumb and index finger are the most affected. Nail changes such as paronychia and onycholysis may be seen. Dermatitis on the face, arms, and genitals has also been reported.[9] Prevention of tulip-driven ACD can be very difficult. The allergen α-methylene-γ-butyrolactone readily penetrates polyvinyl gloves, and also to some extent, latex and neoprene gloves. Nitrile gloves or 4H Silver Shield laminate gloves offer the best protection.[25,26]

Alstroemeria species share the α-methylene-γ-butyrolactone (tulipalin A) allergen. Peruvian lily and Inca lily are common names for *Alstroemeria*. The *Alstroemeria* is a popular flower in the florist industry because of its beautiful shape, variety, year-round availability, and long-lasting nature. Florists may develop chronic fissured dermatitis on the finger tips similar to that seen with tulip fingers. Depigmentation has also been reported at sites of dermatitis and positive patch test sites.[13]

The narcissus (more commonly referred to as daffodil) is a member of the Amaryllidaceae family and is another bulbous plant that may cause ACD. The flowers have a strong scent and can be grown in greenhouses during the winter months. The oil may be harvested and used in the cosmetic, fragrance, and homeopathic industries.[23] The bulb contains an abundance of needle-shaped calcium oxalate crystals that can cause irritant dermatitis. Workers who pick and pack daffodils may develop what has been termed "daffodil itch." On examination, patients may have erythema with somewhat urticarial-appearing papules or more typical eczematous dermatitis. Affected sites may include the hands, face, arms, and genital skin. The hands may look identical to that seen in tulip fingers. Flushing of the face, eye irritation, and headaches have been reported and were attributed to a fragrance component.[23,27,28] The exact hapten that induces ACD is not known.

The hyacinth is another bulbous plant that has been reported to cause ACD. It is a spring-flowering plant, which like daffodils can be grown in the greenhouse and is primarily cultivated for its fragrance. Similar to daffodils, the bulb is high is calcium oxalate crystals. "Hyacinth itch" is the term given to ICD in workers caused from handling hyacinth bulbs.[23,29] The clinical manifestations may be similar to tulip fingers and daffodil itch noted previously. The hapten that causes sensitization and ACD is not known, but could be phenylacetaldehyde, which is also known as hyacinthine.[3]

Garlic (*Allium sativum L.*) is a bulbous member of the Alliaceae plant family. Chives (*Allium schoenoprasum L.*) and the onion (*Allium cepa L.*) are also members of Alliaceae. Garlic, chives, and onions are used primarily as a food source but may also be found in homeopathic treatments. Although growers may develop dermatitis, it is primarily those who use these plants in cooking that are affected by skin disease.[23] The prototypical clinical finding is hyperkeratotic and fissured dermatitis, affecting the first 3 fingers on the nondominant hand. The causative haptens in garlic ACD are felt to be the sulfur compounds allicin and diallyl disulfide and it does not appear that there is significant cross reactivity among garlic, chives, and onions. Allicin is also responsible in large part for garlic's unique smell.[3]

Compositae Plants

Compositae (also called Asteraceae) is a very large family of flowering plants with more than 25,000 species of horticultural plants, weeds and wild flowers, and edible plants.[30] **Table 3** shows some of the more commonly encountered Compositae members. Small tubular flowers tightly arranged on a central capitulum is characteristic (**Fig. 3**). Compositae dermatitis may progress to photosensitivity and chronic actinic dermatitis (CAD) or erythroderma. The cause of the photosensitivity and potential progression to CAD is not known.[31] CAD associated with Compositae sensitivity is clinically the same as that of idiopathic CAD: chronic lichenified dermatitis affecting the exposed areas of the face, V-neck, dorsal arms, and hands. Patients may have improvement in the winter and men older than 40 who live in rural areas and work outdoors are more often affected.

Chrysanthemums ("mums") are decorative members of the Compositae family widely used

Table 3 Compositae family		
Artichoke	Dandelion	Sagebrush
Aster	Endive	Sneezeweed
Black-eyed Susan	Feverfew	Stinkweed
Butterweed	Fleabane	Sunflower
Chamomile	Goldenrod	Tansy
Chicory	Ironweed	Tarragon
Chrysanthemum	Lettuce	Thistle
Cocklebur	Marigold	Tickweed
Cornflower	Pyrethrum	Wormwood
Daisy	Ragweed	Yarrow
Dahlia	Ragwort	Zinnia

Adapted from Crounse RG. Plant dermatitis due to the Compositae (Asteraceae) family. J Am Acad Dermatol 1980;2(5):420; with permission.

in horticulture. They are particularly popular in the fall. *Chrysanthemum indicum L.* and *Chrysanthemum morifolium Ram.* are the most frequently reported to cause ACD, with the leaves and flowers being the most sensitizing parts. The haptens responsible for sensitization are sesquiterpene lactones. As noted previously, erythema and scaling on the face, neck, and upper chest in an airborne pattern is characteristic.

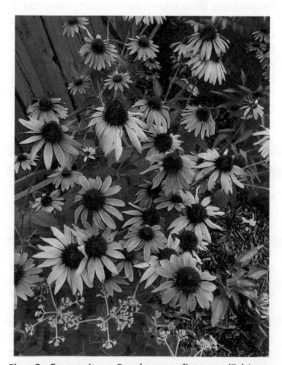

Fig. 3. Compositae Purple coneflowers (Echincea purpurea).

Primrose

Primula obconica is a popular winter-blooming potted plant native to China. The broad leaves are covered with sharp hairs rich in oleoresin, and the flower is described as gobletlike. The plant will continuously bloom during the growing season as long as it is deadheaded. The main sensitizing hapten is primin, which is also known as 2-methoxy-6-pentylbenzoquinone.[3,31] Primin content is the highest from April to August.[32] Patients with primula dermatitis often have edematous to papulovesicular lesions on the fingertips, dorsal fingers, and hands. The lesions may be more likely to show a characteristic streaky or linear eruption similar to that of rhus dermatitis. As noted with the other forms of phytodermatitis, the eyelids, face, and neck may become secondarily involved. Cross reactivity has been reported to occur between *Primula* and tropical woods, such as rosewood.[3,33] *Primula* is also reported to cause conjunctivitis, keratitis, and iritis.

Hardwood Trees

Trees are often overlooked when considering phytodermatitis, but the timber industry employs more than 13.2 million people worldwide and many others work with lumber in carpentry, flooring, and construction.[34] Certain hardwoods are particularly known for the potential for skin disease. *Dalbergia nigra* (also known as Brazilian rosewood or Jacaranda) is a tall tree native to Brazil. It is a valued wood for high-quality furniture and cabinet making. It has also long been considered a superior wood in both looks and sound for guitar making. In 1992, Brazilian rosewood was added to the Convention on International Trade in Endangered Species (CITES) treaty, which strictly banned its exportation. The hapten of *D nigra* is R-4-methoxydalbergione, which is a potent sensitizer. Although this wood is coveted by woodworkers and fine furniture makers, it is also well known to be the cause of severe allergic reactions among these makers.

Softwood Trees (Conifers)

The pine family (Pinaceae) is the most well-known source of softwood. Members of the pine family are trees or shrubs with needle-shaped evergreen leaves. Pine trees are cultivated and harvested for lumber used in construction and home projects. The bulk of lumber sold to consumers at home stores for DIY projects is pine. Colophony (also called rosin) is derived from pine and is a mixture of more than 100 compounds. It is felt that oxidized abietic acid components of this mixture contain the

primary sensitizing haptens.[35] Uses for colophony are vast and diverse, including varnishes, paint driers, printing inks, wax depilatories, cements, soaps, paper, lubricants, tires, plastics, cosmetics, linoleum, chewing gum, and stringing instrument rosin.[3] Turpentine is an oleoresin derived from pine trees and may also act as a sensitizing hapten.[3] Similar to colophony, it is the oxidized (hydroperoxide-containing) form that is allergenic. Turpentine may be used as a solvent in hand cleaners, furniture polishes, paints and thinners, and lacquers. It should also be considered when evaluating contact allergy from essential oils.[36]

Essential Oils

A complete review of essential oils is beyond the scope of this article. Anton de Groot has recently published an excellent series of articles in the journal *Dermatitis* for a more in-depth study of this topic.[36–41] A few important essential oils that are derived from evergreens and are relevant to highlight here include ylang-ylang oil and sandalwood oil. Ylang-ylang (*Cananga odorata*) is an evergreen tree that produces yellowish green flowers that blossom throughout the year. The flowers have a sweet perfume widely desired for their fragrance. Ylang-ylang oil is mainly used in the fragrance industry for floral fragrances but it may also be used as a flavoring agent in beverages, ice cream, candies, chewing gum, and baked goods.[41] Occupational ACD in aromatherapists and massage therapists have been reported.[42,43] Sandalwood (*Santalum album, Santalum spicatum, Santalum austrocaledonicum*) is a small evergreen tree from which a woody sweet-scented essential oil is obtained from the heartwood. Sandalwood oils are widely used in aromatherapy. In addition to being used for its essential oil, sandalwood is used in furniture making.[3] Both ylang-ylang and sandalwood have been reported to cause pigmented ACD associated with cosmetics.

Myroxylon pereirae

Myroxylon pereirae is a tall evergreen tree that grows primarily in Central and South America. Balsam of Peru is a natural viscous material that comes from fresh cuts of *Myroxylon pereirae*. The balsam is a chemically complex mixture of potential allergens, including cinnamates, eugenol, vanillin, benzoic acid derivatives, and coniferin derivatives.[44] It is known for its pleasant cinnamon to vanilla fragrance and flavor. Chemically related compounds are widely used in pharmaceutical preparations and the fragrance industry and therefore balsam of Peru is a good screening test for fragrance and flavoring allergy.[3,45] ACD to balsam of Peru may be seen complicating leg ulcers or in patients reacting to cosmetics or the flavoring in their toothpaste or beverages.

Phytophotodermatitis

Photocontact dermatitis may be either allergic or irritant (phototoxic) in nature. As is always the case, irritant reactions are more common. In fact, the term phytophotodermatitis is generally used to mean the phototoxic reaction that is related to plant furocoumarin content. UV light in the spectrum of 315 nm to 375 nm is the action spectrum for furocoumarins, with the peak spectrum being 330 nm to 335 nm.[46] Plant families known for containing furocoumarins include Apiaceae (Umbelliferae), Rutaceae, and Moraceae.

Apiaceae can be identified by their umbrellalike cluster of long stalks radiating from a central point and include parsley, celery, carrot, fennel, parsnip, and hogweed.[31] The term "stimmer rash or dermatitis" refers to phytophotodermatitis resulting from furocoumarin exposure via a handheld powered rotary tool, such as string trimmers and brush cutters. These tools were previously referred to as strimmers. Members of the Apiaceae family, such as hogweed or wild parsnip, may be encountered and trimmed, resulting in a slinging type of exposure to the plant oils containing furocoumarin.

Rutaceae typically are shrubs or trees that produce fresh fruit. Members of this family include limes, bergamot, rue, bitter orange, lemon, grapefruit, and mokihana. Rue (Ruta graveolens) has been used for centuries as a mosquito repellant by picking the fruit, crushing it in your hands, and rubbing the resulting material on your skin. Several cases of photophytodermatitis have been reported to result from this practice.[47] Mokihana is frequently used in Hawaiian leis. The fig tree is a member of Moraceae. Clinical reactions may range from simple erythematous lesions or hyperpigmentation to robust bullous lesions. Unlike allergic reactions, pruritus is not typically a dominant symptom. Berloque pigmented dermatitis due to a perfume, lotion or other cosmetic containing furocoumarins is the most well-known cause of hyperpigmented phototoxic eruptions.

Photoallergic contact dermatitis from plants is uncommon. Photoallergic reactions have been reported to musk ambrette in aftershave lotions,[48] sandalwood oil, diallyl disulfide, alantolactone, Arnica montana, sesquiterpene lactone, pyrethrum, and Tanacetum vulgare.[49]

Patch Testing

The gold standard for the diagnosis of ACD is patch testing. The Thin-layer Rapid Use Epicutaneous (T.R.U.E. TEST) patch test is the only system that is currently available that has approval from the Food and Drug Administration for patch testing. It is indicated for the diagnosis of ACD in patients 6 years of age and older. With respect to evaluation of phytodermatitis, the T.R.U.E. TEST contains 3 screening allergens: colophony, balsam of Peru, and parthenolide. It is important to understand that this is a very limited evaluation and that full evaluation of suspected phytodermatitis will typically require more expanded testing. Expanded standardized test substances can be ordered from patch test vendors such as Chemotechnique Diagnostics and allergEAZE. It is important to keep in mind that it is never advisable to perform patch testing to unknown plants or substances. Many plants have the potential to cause strong or even severe irritant or allergic reactions.

REFERENCES

1. Botanic Gardens Conservation International. [Online] Available at: https://www.bgci.org/policy/1521/. Accessed September 1, 2019.
2. Chou M, Mikhaylov D, Lazic Struger T. Moisturizers: A comparison based on allergens and economic value. Dermatitis 2018;29:339–44.
3. Benezra C. Plant contact dermatitis. Philadelphia: B.C. Decker Inc; 1985.
4. Modi GM, Doherty CB, Katta R, et al. Irritant contact dermatitis from plants. Dermatitis 2009;20:63–78.
5. Bowers AG. Phytophotodermatitis. Am J Contact Dermatitis 1999;10:89–93.
6. Freeman K, Hubbard SH, Warin AP. Strimmer rash. Contact Dermatitis 1984;10:117–8.
7. Elpern DJ, Mitchell JC. Phytophotodermatitis from mokihana fruits in Hawaiian lei. Contact Dermatitis 1984;10:224–6.
8. Martin H, Martin CH. Causticite du Dieffenbachia picta. Cah Med Lyon 1977;3:869.
9. Stoner JG, Rasmussen JE. Plant dermatitis. J Am Acad Dermatol 1983;9(1):1–15.
10. Kohen SG. Seasonal ragweed dermatitis: association of immediate and delayed types of pollen sensitivity. Arch Dermatol 1959;79:328–33.
11. Fisher A. Contact dermatitis. 2. Philadelphia: Lea & Febiger; 1978. p. 243–72.
12. Klingman AM. Poison ivy (Rhus) dermatitis. Arch Dermatol 1958;77:149.
13. Marks JG, Elsner P, DeLeo V. Contact & occupational dermatology. 3rd edition. St Louis (MO): Mosby; 2002.
14. Kadlubowska D, Bargman H, Sasseville D. Systemic contact dermatitis caused by inhaled cashew oil smoke. Contact Dermatitis 2016;75:240–59.

15. Reginella R, Fairfield J, Marks J. Hyposensitization to poison ivy after working in a cashew nut shell oil processing factory. Contact Dermatitis 1989;20(4):274–9.

16. Nogueira Diógenes MJ, Oliveira Ramos FD, Alencar Oliveira AD, et al. Paronychia in cashew nut industry workers. Contact Dermatitis 2002;47(2):121.

17. Mason HS. The toxic principles of poison ivy. III. The structure of bhilawanol. J Am Chem Soc 1945;67:418–20.

18. Oka A, Saito F, Yasuhara T, et al. A study of cross-reactions between mango contact allergens and urushiol. Contact Dermatitis 2004;51(5–6):292–6.

19. Zakon SJ. Contact dermatitis due to mango. JAMA 1939;113:1808.

20. Kim A, Christiansen S. Mango: pulp fiction? Contact Dermatitis 2015;73(2):123–4.

21. Hassan I, Rasool F, Akhtar S, et al. Contact dermatitis caused by tulips: identification of contact sensitizers in tulip workers of Kashmir Valley in North India. Contact Dermatitis 2018;78(1):64–9.

22. Mijnssen V. Pathogenesis and causative agent of "tulip finger. Br J Dermatol 1969;81:737–45.

23. Bruynzeel DP. Bulb dermatitis. Contact Dermatitis 1997;37:70–7.

24. Overton S. Dermatitis from handling flower bulbs. Lancet 1926;2:1003.

25. Marks FG. Allergic contact dermatitis to Alstromeria. Arch Dermatol 1988;124:914–6.

26. De Haan P. Prevention of contact dermatitis due to tulipalin A. Barcelona (Spain): Abstract Book ESCD; 1994. p. 11.

27. Walsh D. Investigation of dermatitis amongst flower-pickers in the Scilly Islands, the so-called lily rash. Br Med J 1910;(2):851–6.

28. Palmer WH. "Lily rash": an occupational dermatitis. Lancet 1934;(2):755–6.

29. Freeman WT. A note on the skin irritation caused by handling hyacinth bulbs. Br J Dermatol 1897;9:66–7.

30. Fowler J, Zirwas M. Fisher's contact dermatitis. 7th edition. Phoenix (AZ): Walsworth; 2019.

31. Sasseville D. Clinical patterns of phytodermatitis. Dermatol Clin 2009;27:299–308.

32. Hjorth N. Seasonal variations in contact dermatitis. Acta Derm Venereol 1967;47(6):409–18.

33. Mitchell JC, Rook A. Botanical dermatology. Vancouver (Canada): Greengrass; 1979. p. 554–67.

34. The World Bank. Available at: https://www.world bank.org/en/topic/forests/brief/forests-generate-jobs-and-incomes. Accessed September 1, 2019.

35. Downs A, Sansom J. Colophony allergy: a review. Contact Dermatitis 1999;41:305–10.

36. de Groot A, Schmidt E. Essential oils, part IV: contact allergy. Dermatitis 2016;27(4):170–5.

37. de Groot AC, Schmidt E. Essential oils, part i: introduction. Dermatitis 2016;27(2):9–42.

38. de Groot A, Schmidt E. Part II: general aspects. Dermatitis 2016;27(2):43–9.

39. de Groot AC, Schmidt E. Essential oils, part iii: chemical composition. Dermatitis 2016;27(4):161–9.

40. de Groot A, Schmidt E. Essential oils, part V: peppermint oil, lavender oil, and lemongrass oil. Dermatitis 2016;27(6):325–32.

41. de Groot AC, Schmidt E. Essential oils, part VI: sandalwood oil, ylang-ylang oil, and jasmine absolute. Dermatitis 2017;28(1):14–21.

42. Cockayne SE, Gawkrodger. Occupational contact dermatitis in an aromatherapist. Contact Dermatitis 1997;37(6):306–7.

43. Bleasel N, Tate B, Rademaker M. Allergic contact dermatitis following exposure to essential oils. Australas J Dermatol 2002;43(3):211–3.

44. Hausen B. Identification of new allergenic constituents and proof of evidence for coniferyl benzoate in balsam of Peru. Am J Contact Dermat 1995;6(4):199–208.

45. Scheman A, Rakowski EM, Chou V, et al. Balsam of Peru: past and future. Dermatitis 2013;24(4):153–60.

46. Carlsen K, Weismann K. Phytodermatitis in 19 children admitted to hospital and their differential diagnoses: child abuse and herpes simplex virus infection. J Am Acad Dermatol 2007;57(9):S88–91.

47. Eickhorst K, DeLeo V, Csaposs J. Rue the herb: *Ruta graveolens*-associated phytophototoxicity. Dermatitis 2007;18(1):51–5.

48. Kroon S. Musk Ambrette, a new cosmetic sensitizer and photosensitizer. Contact Derm 1979;5:337–8.

49. Victor F, Cohen D, Sorter N. A 20-year analysis of previous and emerging allergens that elicit photoallergic contact dermatitis. J Am Acad Dermatol 2010;62(4):605–10.

Moving?

Make sure your subscription moves with you!

To notify us of your new address, find your **Clinics Account Number** (located on your mailing label above your name), and contact customer service at:

Email: journalscustomerservice-usa@elsevier.com

800-654-2452 (subscribers in the U.S. & Canada)
314-447-8871 (subscribers outside of the U.S. & Canada)

Fax number: 314-447-8029

Elsevier Health Sciences Division
Subscription Customer Service
3251 Riverport Lane
Maryland Heights, MO 63043

*To ensure uninterrupted delivery of your subscription, please notify us at least 4 weeks in advance of move.

ELSEVIER

Printed and bound by CPI Group (UK) Ltd, Croydon, CR0 4YY

03/10/2024

01040374-0017